LOSING ONE HUNDRED POUNDS

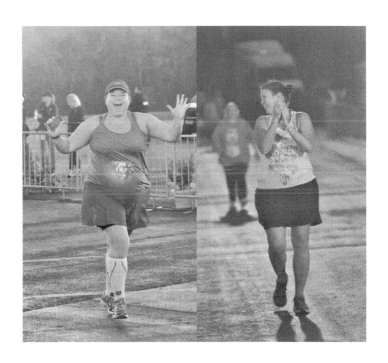

By
Clara Boyd
LETTING GO of so much more than just the weight

CONTENTS

Losing One Hundred Pounds	
My Thoughts	1
Introduction	4
LIFE BEFORE LETTING GO	5
LETTING GO OF 13.1	11
LETTING GO OF THE WEIGHT	49
LETTING GO OF CONTROL	66
LETTING GO THROUGH MUSIC	99
LETTING GO THROUGH PHYSICAL STRENGTH	104
LETTING GO IS A CONSCIOUS EFFORT	116
LETTING GO OF EVERYTHING	120
REFERENCES & PHOTOGRAPGY ACKNOWLEDGEMENTS	124

MY THOUGHTS

No two people will ever be on the same journey – no matter how similar the itinerary may look. Perhaps they are in the same car, listening to the same song, looking at the same foliage on the side of the road. However, their experiences will be different. The same can be said with weight loss journeys.

There are so many weight loss stories out there; what makes this one different from the others? This story is my story; a snippet of my journey. Take it for what it's worth. This book is a collection of my journal posts on social media, my private journals before, during, and after my weight loss, as well as a recollection of thought regarding those posts. It is emotional; my personal feelings and opinions. It is honest and raw, sad and funny. It is ME.

At the time of press, I am not a spokesman for any of the products mentioned in this book. In fact, OPTIFAST is a registered trademark of Société des Produits Nestlé S.A., Vevey, Switzerland. No endorsement by Nestlé is implied or intended, and no sponsorship or support was provided by Nestlé. I quote people in this book, as there are some smart people in this world. Brilliant people actually, so why not pass along their knowledge to you? I also happen to mention the name of some famous places and landmarks in this book. You know what? This is real life - I went to some real places, including Walt Disney World, and their various properties and events worldwide.

This is not a diet plan. <u>Please seek medical assistance if you are wanting to lose weight, or change your lifestyle.</u> I am not a nutritionist, nor do I claim to be a medical professional who can assist you in this type of lifestyle change. The only advice that I will give you is that if you plan on starting any type of program – research it, research it a second time, and then a third time.

Dedication

This book is dedicated to the friends and family that were supportive of this project, that kept it positive but realistic, and stuck around, even when I told cheesy jokes, blurted out useless trivia, or sang a Barry Manilow tune or two.

To my friends – To Val, Leigh, Carol, Odalis, Vivian, Kelley, Laura, Robyn, Trish, Vince, Mike M, Autumn, Mike C, Colton, Brad, Taylor, Mrs. Stevens. Thank you for your contributions reading the many drafts, bouncing ideas with me, crying with me, laughing with me, and letting me tell my story. In your own way, each one of you have encouraged me to be successful. This journey started all because I was at a donut shop on Cape Cod drinking coffee on my 42nd birthday when Val stated, "Clara – this is YOUR year!" While sitting there I was reminded that Vivian, a close friend, told me I needed to take all of my journal entries and turn them into a book. As I sat at the airport waiting for my plane home, I searched through the available online books on how to write a book. I needed to find something to read for the trip back to Florida, and I thought – who the hell would actually buy a book this idiotic? You know who? Me! And before I knew it – I was putting the finishing touches on the book.

To my family – Kim – There is no one else I would want as my big sister. Thank you for paving the way for me. THAT'S MY SISTER! Rob – you are my favorite brother-in-law! You were the perfect addition to our family. I appreciate the two of you for giving me the best presents ever – Taylor and Alex. They are my favorites. To Taylor and Alex – it is true – you are my favorites. Thank you for giving me the best name I could ever imagine – Aunt. Be

Clara Boyd

courageous, be brave, be the strong women inside and out that I know you are – that is what makes you beautiful. 1-4-3 & WMW? FOREVER!

To my parents, Bob and Nancy. Thank you for everything you do for me on a daily basis. I am so glad that God made me your daughter. And thank you for not trading me in for the other baby in the nursery like you always joked about when I was little.

Finally, to everyone that bought this book – Thank YOU! If you ever have that idea that you believe is just a crazy dream – go for it. I did, and you are about to start reading it. Right now.

INTRODUCTION

I am staring out into the rainforest of Alaska on an afternoon in June. It is 50 degrees and misty, but I am sweating, and my mouth is dry as the desert in Death Valley, California. My mind is racing – will the cable hold me? Will I plummet down through the trees to land on the jagged rocks below? There is no way I can do this – my feet are not going to be on a platform. I need my feet to be on a solid surface. I know I have lost enough weight that I am under the weight limit, but my nerves are getting the best of me. I cannot let go! I need to be in control. I often think to myself, Clara – you have overcome so much in your life. Just shut up and LET GO. But why can't you?

LIFE BEFORE LETTING GO

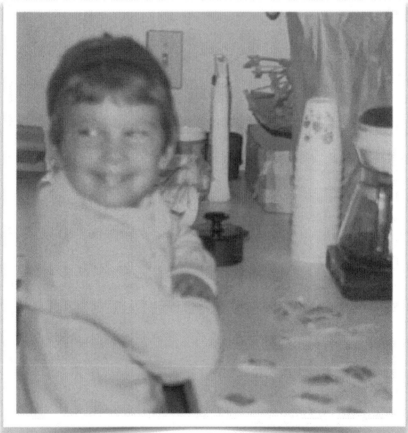

Me in my Brownie Beanie, early 1980s

Losing One Hundred Pounds

My weight problems started on July 13, 1976. I was 8 pounds 8 ounces. They really did not start that day, but I will spare you the obligatory "first bath" picture that every baby born in the 1970s had taken. We all had a huge belly; we had chubby thighs.

We were children of baby boomers; grandchildren of WWII veterans. What did that mean? We all had cereal for breakfast; lunch was a sandwich, chips, and fruit; and dinner - we finished what was on our plate, which consisted of a meat, starch, vegetable, and sometimes a dessert. If you didn't finish it, you sat there until you did. You did chores around the house and were held accountable for your actions and the actions of your friends.

I was the biggest female of growing up in my classes. Looking back now, I should have known – Dutch women are tall! My genetics were going to predispose me to be on the back row of every class picture. There was never an option to join the rest of the girls in the front of the picture. My first memory of feeling insecure about my weight was in fifth grade. One of the boys in the class said his weight out loud - 114 pounds. I thought… that is how much I weigh! He immediately said – "I am so fat!" I shrunk down as far as I could in my seat, thinking – if he thinks he is fat at that weight, then that must mean I am fat too. I knew I was always taller than all the other girls, which naturally meant I was bigger, but I never thought – I must be fat. Now I feel the need to add here that I have been 6-foot-tall since 7th grade. That is the year that I had scoliosis surgery where, one my back was straightened out, I grew 8 inches in height. If middle school was not awkward enough, imagine you leave your 7th grade year for hospital homebound already taller than all the boys, and you come back 8th grade year 6 feet tall! Let the nicknames start… Sasquatch, Bigfoot, you name it – Ugh! This was the first time in my life I felt so insecure that I just wanted to not go to school. I was so self-conscious. I was 147 pounds, and I knew at 6 feet tall I was so fat, I was disgusting.

During this time in my life, I should have enjoyed going to the

6

mall shopping and hanging out. All the cool kids did it. However, growing up, there was not a big and tall store for teenage girls. When I was in high school I was a size 12/14 and the rest of my friends were a size 2/4. Compared to all of my friends, I thought I was huge! I did not want to go to the mall, I was too embarrassed. I wish I could go back now and tell my younger self to be proud – Screw what other people thought!

I was on the Flag squad all four years in high school. Trying on my flag uniform for the fitting was stressful, and I feared this day every year. Girls would adjust the uniform every year, and so they were not true to size. I was always scared I would not fit into the largest skirt. What would I do if I did not fit into the skirt? I needed be able to fit into a uniform to be on the squad, and I knew that ordering a larger size was not an option.

School dances always stressed me out. I was always worried I would never find a dress that would fit me. While I always did find one, there were times we went to multiple stores before we could find one. My mom always made sure we could find one. I look back now as an adult and can't thank her enough. She must have known the fear I had that I would not find a dress that would fit. What would I do? How times have changed. My largest size in high school was a size 14. Thank goodness society acknowledges that women are larger than a size 14 now; and these women want to be fashionable too!

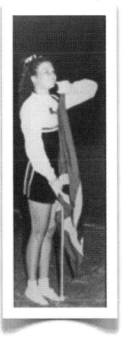

Me, my sophomore year in high school. I thought I was huge.

How distorted were our body images of ourselves when we were teens?

To be that fit again would be amazing! (Sarasota High School Yearbook, Sailor's Log 1992)

In college I truly did find the freshmen fifteen as they like to say, plus some. Clemson University is an agricultural college, so there was a dairy on campus with fresh ice cream, and the best blue cheese around! I discovered beer, and late-night eating. I also found that mak- ing egg sandwiches for friends after a night of drinking was my forte. Everyone knew that egg sandwiches were being made at S1E (my apartment) at 2 am. The social aspect of college was great, but earning my degree was my main priority, and I received a degree in Health Education. I have the knowledge, just not the willpower to follow it, especially in college.

I earned my second degree at University of North Florida in Jacksonville. While the partying subsided a little bit, my life started to revolve around my classes and clinicals. I was studying Sports Medicine – Athletic Training. Earning this degree was very intense, as are many medical degrees. The group of students in the program not only took classes together, but we spent the majority of all waking hours together. We ate around athletic events. The most memorable was during college football Saturdays. Before we would go to take the field for pregame, we would drop a few packages of hotdogs (still in the plastic) and a can of chili into the hydrocollators (the machine that holds the hot water and hot packs) On top of the hydrocollator we would place the hot dog buns to warm them. During halftime, while we were tending to the injured athletes, someone – typically a lower classman, would prepare hotdogs for everyone. On the way out the door, you would grab a hot-dog and eat it on your way back into the game. In addition, we were eating a lot of fast food and there were late nights as we were studying for national boards, and still enjoying a few nights of blowing off steam.

After my two bachelors, I decided to get my third degree – my Master's at Florida State University, in Sports Management. In the years' time I received this degree, I also was the head athletic trainer for an Arena 2 Football team and started working at a local high school as their athletic trainer and teacher. With very little sleep, and eating with professional football players on the road, I started gaining weight at a very quick pace. After that year ended, I remained at the high school for approximately 10 more years; working 14-hour days, as a teacher/athletic trainer. I would eat meals when I could – usually concession stand food, fast food, or late at night when I got home. I lived alone and did not want to cook meals for one. It was just easier to eat out. I was too tired to work out when I got home, so I was truly living a sedentary lifestyle. Ironically, I was teaching the health courses and Anatomy & Physiology. Talk about do as I say, and not as I do!

This sedentary lifestyle plus hypothyroidism and polycystic ovarian syndrome snowballed into me having pre-diabetic insulin resistance, high cholesterol, and high blood pressure, and weighing 326 pounds. Wait. What? 326 pounds – How did I get there? I have heard people verbalize about others – "They are so large; how did they get THAT BIG?" Trust me
– Life happens, and then one day you wake up, 326 pounds. You don't want to gain weight, or get THAT BIG. My life was spinning out of control. I had to stop it.

I ended up leaving the brick and mortar educational world and transitioned to the virtual world, and have been there since. The career change will allow for me to schedule in time for the gym, a break in the afternoon to go for a walk, time to cook healthy meals at home – this will be great! I will be able to finally make ME a priority! You would think that means with this newfound gift of time I would put me first, until old habits return...

LETTING GO OF 13.1

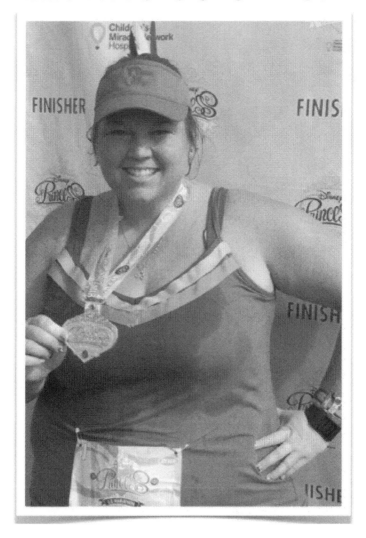

There are many times in my life that I would make a promise to myself and would break it. We all do it, and it is usually on January 1st around midnight. How many times is there a New Year's resolution that is busted by the first weekend of the new year? Lose weight; Eat better; you know the resolutions. You may even give it the old college try to make it to the gym for three weeks, and then it tapers off. Life gets in the way – how many times did that happen to me? More than I would like to admit. When I turned 39, I knew I was going to complete a half marathon by the time I turned 40. Being a Disney fanatic, there is only one place I was going to complete this goal – Walt Disney World in Orlando, of course! (If you plan to run a race, be it a 5K, or a marathon – Disney puts on one helluva race!). While some people may wear typical race gear, some people dress up like characters, other people will dress for the theme of the race. The theme of this half marathon was the Princess Half Marathon. Being a Clemson Tiger, I knew exactly who I would be…. Tiger Lily from *Peter Pan* of course!

I had completed a few 5Ks in my day, but never something as daunting as a half marathon. In the running world, the joke is that people that participate in half marathons are only half crazy. Let me just say – **no one that runs races is crazy. They are all brave and amazing!**

I signed up for the race with three amazing ladies. Two of the ladies live here locally in Tallahassee, FL, and one lives in Key Largo, FL. Training looks a little different in Key Largo I am sure – beaches, palm trees, coconuts; where in Tallahassee it is more like southern Georgia – rolling hills, Georgia red clay, and oak trees. Many days there were deer on our training runs that would watch us, making sure we did not get too close. I wondered if they watched us and were laughing at us speculating why we're running and not driving in a car like the rest of the humans. To keep each other accountable with our training, as well as en- courage each other, I started a private Facebook group called PHM (Princess Half Marathon) for the four of us.

October 20, 2015 - PHM

Clara Boyd

Let the Royal Training Begin! Princess Half Marathon training started this morning. Which meant, last night I was too nervous to sleep! I will not be the fastest, or the most impressive runner in the race, but I will be the most impressive me ever! :)

Matthew 19:26 "With man this is impossible, but with God all things are possible."

October 22, 2015 - PHM

Good morning my Princesses! Day 2 of running for the week. Make sure to get 30 minutes in today. Laura got new running shoes this week. Nice pair of Brooks! I know you broke them in yesterday. Great job! Cindy did her 30 minutes on Tuesday with an average pace of 12 min/mile. You are doing awesome! And Carol ran half of a half. I am so jelly of you - and so proud at the same time. Check in here once you run today. I am doing my 30 on the "dreadmill". I mean treadmill. I will be at the gym anyway, so we will see how this goes.
Happy Running!

October 22, 2015 – Facebook

I did my 30 minutes running this morning. I decided to do it on the dreadmill. I have a love/hate relationship with that thing. I love it when I am done, but I surely hate it while running on it. I will confess - I am so graceful, that I am worried I will trip. I will be that person in the gym, face down on the ground with the treadmill still going. So, I went a little slower of a pace, completed the 30 minutes and then went right into an arms workout with my trainer. So, what does this mean? This means I have no use of my legs or my arms today. Lord help me if I have to move. Happy Thursday!!!!

October 24, 2015 – PHM

Distance: 2.01 miles

Time: 36:57

Pace: 18:20 min/mile

Good morning ladies! This Tiger Lily is exhausted! Today is 2 miles we need to run. Just finished mine. I only ran for about 2 minutes of this as my asthma kicked in pretty quick. Walked the rest of the way. Refused to stop. However, with the Mile 10 ramp in mind, I chose to walk the huge hill at the end of this instead of going down another street which would have been flat. So - while my time is not the best, I find pride in the fact I finished strong. Let's hear from you when you finish yours today :)

At 326 pounds, I had exercise-induced asthma. It is astounding to look back on this post. I remember sitting in the allergy and asthma doctor's office when he diagnosed me. I went primarily as I believed I was having asthma symptoms, but they ran all the tests, stuck me so many times, tested me for every allergen, and it came back I was allergic to dog saliva and grass, and exercise induced asthma. So, I am overweight, but I cannot exercise. I have an inside dog, but I cannot workout outside. Awesome. Even better than that, if you remember, in my previous life, I was an athletic trainer – I lived my life outside on football fields! That explains my constant life of sinusitis. I digress. The doctor was an older gentleman who was trying to explain to me that the asthma would get better if I lost weight. He was politely trying to explain that I was big chested and that the weight of my breasts pressing down on my lungs was intensifying the asthma. Catch 22. Two different types of inhalers later, I start to workout...

October 27, 2015 – PHM

Happy Tuesday! It is raining here :(How is the weather in Key Largo??? We need to be like the post office. No matter the weather... We have to get the run in. I did it on a treadmill. Thought for the day - what if it is raining during the race? We have to be ready, and there will not be a treadmill there for us to run on. So - next time it rains - I am running in it. Have an awesome run today!!!

Clara Boyd

This was something that kept me up at night. What if it did rain during the race? What was I going to do? I am Type A. I need to be in control! This CANNOT happen! I want to have perfect race weather. If it rains, I may slip and fall. If it rains, there will be mud, which will be harder to run in. I should change what I will wear. A visor. I will wear a hat or a visor to keep the rain out of my eyes – that is what I will do... (Breathe, Clara, Breathe...)

October 27, 2015 – Facebook

Where are the sweeps? I have heard so many different stories of where they are - including a final one as you are coming into EPCOT. I am training to stay under 15 min/mile; but for my sanity, if anyone has a list of them, that would be greatly appreciated.
Thanks :)

Have I mentioned I was Type A?

October 29, 2015 – PHM

Happy Thursday! Shout out to you if you ran today! I know Cindy kicked it in gear already :) Mom had surgery this morning, so I only walked a very slow mile. I will run in the morning. Looking forward to hearing about your running!!!

I found out very fast at this point that life can start creeping into training schedules. Just like anything in life, there can always be an excuse. Don't let the excuse find its way in there. Let your goal be bigger than your excuse!

October 31, 2015 - Facebook

I truly dislike the 'bathroom selfie'. But I had to show you how HAPPY I am after a 5K practice run in my Sparkle Skirt! I will be wearing this next week at Disney and wanted to run in it to make sure I could do it. Why did I ever doubt a Sparkle Skirt???? I promise you - this was the best decision ever!!! Side note... I have asthma, and my inhaler fit easily into the pocket and was accessible during my run! This skirt is amazing!!!!

Oh, the bathroom selfie! I will never understand it – maybe because I cannot perfect it. Maybe because I do not need to see someone's toilet, or someone's toothbrush where they did not rinse off the toothpaste. Who knows? Anyway – This was in response to a company named "Sparkle Skirts". Being 326 pounds, my thighs were rubbing together like two sticks trying to start a camp fire. There was nothing sparkling about them. The chaffing was un- bearable. I was on every blog I could find trying to find plus size workout clothes. (don't worry – I will get on my soap box about that later on...). These skirts are legit. There are leggings underneath them that stay where they are supposed to. For the first time, I had found a product that allowed me to work out and focus on working out. Not taking a few steps and pulling the shorts out of my woman parts! The smile on my face, as cheesy as it is – is real! I am happy I found a running skirt – a PLUS SIZE running skirt! YES - BIG GIRLS RUN!

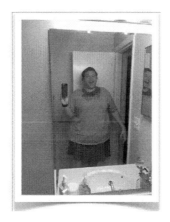

November 2, 2015

I am anxious, but I am starting to feel like I could complete the 5K. I had to travel for work to Orlando for the week (How perfect was that?) So, on that Monday, I packed the car, and headed down with a little confidence that I may just be a-OK! I may just survive this race! I was completing this 5K at Disney merely for the fact

Clara Boyd

that I wanted to see the logistics of a Disney race. (Come on – are you really shocked? If you have read this far into the book, you know I am Type-A, OCD, and have to be in control. Hi my name is Clara, and I am a control freak...)

November 5, 2015 – Facebook

Today I am thankful for hotel gyms. It is not the same as walking with Kelley in the mornings, but it got the job done! I also proudly wore my Clemson/West Virginia Orange Bowl shirt. If you don't know, that is one of Clemson's worst losses in history. But I wear the shirt with pride. Through adversity you find strength and success. Today I will find success!!! (And as always - GO TIGERS!!!)

Oh, this post makes me laugh. Two great things about this post. An amazing friend and Clemson, of course! Kelley is a dear friend – one of those friends that is a sister from an- other mister. If you haven't noticed, I have more of those in my life than not. Those are your true girlfriends, the ones that God put on this Earth for you to find at different times in your life. On January of 2015, we started walking as a New Year's resolution, and that was the first resolution of the sort that I have kept! We keep each other accountable. There is a text every night to make sure that we are walking the next morning, usually initiated by Kelley, and then at o-dark-thirty, we walk 1.5 miles. Just enough time to catch up on the gossip from the day before, and to get our hearts pumping for the day ahead. We both live on the outskirts of Tallahassee, so on our walks we are greeted by deer, rabbits, and other beautiful wildlife. Every so often there is a snake, which gets my heart pumping – and not in a good way! We see the sunrise and have a few moments of peace before the day gets crazy with schedules and work. Getting out of that routine can screw with your day a little bit, and it has been a morning ritual that I look forward to even to this day. On the days that I travel, or for whatever other reason we cannot walk, I feel like my day just did not start off on the right foot. Maybe it is because I am creature of habit.

Losing One Hundred Pounds

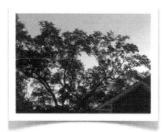

This is a heart that was created by the branches of two trees that Kelley and I see on our walks daily. Clemson played West Virginia in the 2012 Orange Bowl and lost 70-26. In that game, West Virginia became the first team to score 70 points in a bowl game. I used to wear that shirt on days I needed to find extra strength. Clemson is currently a powerhouse in football and that is amazing. However, I went to Clemson in the 1990s and if you know anything about football, you are already laughing. If you do not, let's just say, we were happy in the 1990s if we had a winning season, blessed if we went to a bowl game, and if we beat University of South Carolina? It was a miracle! I cheered for the football team back then just as loudly as I do today! I bleed orange and purple...I have since the day I applied for college in August of 1993, the only university I applied to. I cried tears of joy when I received my acceptance letter in October of 1993 and knew that my heart belonged in Clemson. There is a pride that goes with being a Clemson alumnus. I truly find strength in every win or loss that Clemson has. Thus, that shirt, although now long gone, on the day of that workout provided the strength that I needed. 70-26. Push harder. Go further. Finish strong.

November 6, 2015 - Facebook

This just got real!!!! I will be representing the last corral proudly!

Clara Boyd

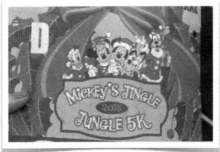
My first runDisney race

OK – for my non-runners out there let me break this down for you. Corral placement is HUGE in a race. This being my first race, my pace that I registered with (or how fast I ran a mile) I was placed in the last corral. Insert shuttering or laughing here for all you runners. You do not want to be in the last corral, typically. As in, if they sweep during the race, you may be swept. What does that mean? If you do not keep a certain pace, the race officials may tell you to stop the race and escort you to the finish line. On this particular Disney 5K, they did not sweep so this was not a concern.

Losing One Hundred Pounds

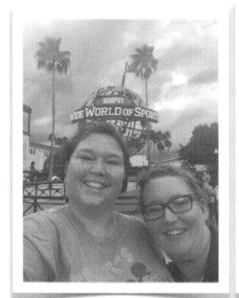 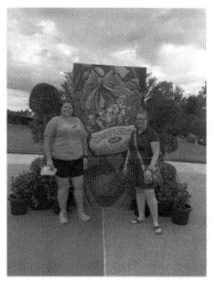

Laura and I absorbed in every aspect of the race expo. Many of the blogs recommend that is this is your first expo that you do not bring your credit cards. Whatever I have total control. Bahahaha! I should have listened. Like a kid in a candy store buying everything I thought I may have possibly needed. I felt like Rene Russo in *Tin Cup* where she had purchased all the products to better her golf game, but insert running gadgets. If you are starting your running journey – trust me on this – LEAVE THE CREDIT CARD AT HOME! Your bank account will thank you!

Clara Boyd

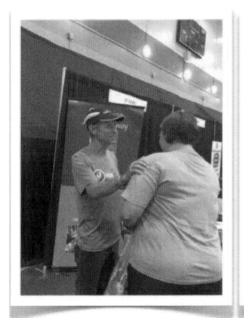 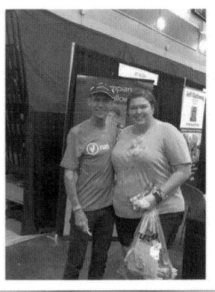

I finally get to meet Jeff Galloway! While the I spent a lot of money at the expo, the best part of the experience was priceless. As we turned the corner we could see Jeff Galloway. Who is Jeff Galloway you may ask? Jeff Galloway is an American Olympian who was on the 1972 US Olympic team, and a lifetime runner. He perfected this interval method of walk/run and has authored many books. In my running journey, I landed upon the Galloway method as it is known and have been using it to complete my training. If you are interested in running, I recommend you find a method that best suits you, but this method is my jam! The basics of the method is that you walk for a certain amount of time, and then run for a certain amount of time; continuing to switch between the two until your mileage has completed. That is a very basic description, and I most certainly do not do it justice. I have found my comfort zone at 40 seconds walk, 40 seconds run. Some walk for 1 minute and run for 4 minutes, but it is really whatever works best for you. Research the method for more information, and to find your comfort zone.

What was more important about this meeting was my humbleness and gratefulness to this man. I am outspoken, and rarely am speechless. I waited in line, as if I was a child waiting to see Santa in December. We were all runners waiting to pay our respect. When it was my turn to speak to him, it was if I was Ralphie in *A Christmas Story* seeing Santa. My mouth opened, but I could not speak. I wanted to tell him so much, but I could not speak. I wanted to tell him, that I had found a courage that I never knew I had in me because of his kindness and guidance. His patience, yet perseverance in the app – this is what I would listen to on my runs. However, nothing came out of my mouth. I could feel the tears streaming down my face, and my lip quivering. This is the point he grabbed my shoulder and told me how proud he was of me for making the change in my life! (WHAT!!!! Jeff Galloway just said he was proud of ME???? Now there was no way those tears were going to stop! I was a blubbering idiot!). I told him I lived in Tallahassee, and that was all I could get out. He reminisced with me about his time at Florida State University, and that is where he met his lovely wife, Barb. I finally calmed down enough to humbly tell him my goal of running the half marathon in February, and that I would be doing so by his method. There was no doubt in his mind – he knew I would do it. That was the confidence that I needed. Jeff Gal-loway believed in me! I can do this!

November 7, 2015

The day of the 5K is here! Laura and I signed up for this race to see the logistics of a Disney race in preparation for the half marathon. Let's be honest, it's Walt Disney World! We are going to be fun! The only problem – Clemson is playing FSU. FSU recently lost their first game of the season, while Clemson was still undefeated – this is going to be an awesome game! If we win this game, we were going to go to the ACC Championship. BYOG was termed by Dabo Sweeney, Clemson's head football coach, after the Auburn game meaning – Bring Your Own Guts. I cannot think of a more fitting T-shirt to wear for the race. It is my first official Disney race, I am anxious, and I am bringing my own guts! I am not at the Clemson game, where my heart is, but I am where I need to be. I am figuring out how the heck the race worked. At the end of the day – I am not going to screw up the half marathon. That is what today is all about. This is business (and a little Disney fun too).

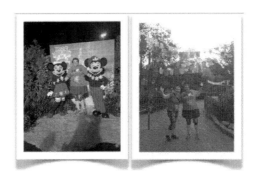

November 7, 2015 – Post 5K

This day was quickly brought much self-doubt. Laura, myself, and one of my other sisters from another mister – Odalis, started the race together. Within two minutes, Odalis was off and running. Running a race has a simple etiquette. Runners are runners. Odalis is a runner. I am not. While it is nice to try to stay together during a race, if someone has a different pace than you, you respect that, and you let them run their race. Laura and I are overall the same pace; well let's be honest. Laura takes more steps, but I just have longer legs. We had our interval pacer app hooked on my shirt and ready to go. We found out fast in the crowd of the last coral, we did not have the ability to use the interval pacer. There was no way to keep any sort of running pace as people were walking everywhere. Imagine a Mardi Gras-sized crowd in the parking lot of Animal Kingdom, shoulder-to-shoulder people trying to start the race. We were not aware we needed go to the left to try to run. We were race novices, and it showed! I started verbalizing quickly to Laura how disappointed I was in myself for not being able to run. The size of the crowd was giving me anxiety, and it was overpowering my thoughts and confidence in my abilities to complete the race. Due to the anxiety, I could not control my breathing, and thus I could not run. It is a bit overwhelming the first time.

During the race, I found myself behind this woman, and it made me take a moment to breathe. I loved her shirt. DLF > DNF > DNS. It read "Dead Last Finish is greater than Did Not Finish, which is greater than Did Not Start". Thank you, God! I needed a sign! I shut my trap and learned to enjoy the moment! Now, being inspired by her, I tried to keep pace with her, but she eventually lost us, because she was so amazing, but I am so glad I took a picture of her shirt. When we finished the 5K, another race participant came up and congratulated me. Upon chatting she mentioned that she heard me telling Laura during the race how I doubted myself. She told me to stop doubting myself and encouraged me. Talk about inspiring! Runners really are cool people!

November 7, 2015 – Facebook

Post from Mom

Proud of Clara, Laura, and Odalis all completed the Disney run this morning

Mom has always been my rock… even if she would not miss the Clemson game for my first Disney race. Hey – at least she has her priorities straight. Go Tigers!

November 8, 2015 – Facebook

*Finished Disney's Jingle Jungle in true BOTP fashion yesterday. But it was great as it allowed me to analyze what I still needed to do for my training for the Princess Half Marathon in February. I walked a lot more than I thought I would, and a dear friend stayed right by my side. I don't remember exactly what I said but it was something negative about my abilities (I was freaking out a little **about not being able to*** *physically run during the intervals like I trained to do). After the race another runner came up to me and acknowledged my comments and told me I did great - don't let the negative thoughts get in my mind. That was so nice of her, and it meant so much to me. Runners are so positive, so encouraging, so supportive, and BOTP is the greatest place to be during a race. Good luck to all BOTPers in your races today!!!*

Looking back, BOTP – Back of the Pack – it really is not a bad place to be at all! Just as long as you know how to maneuver it. Remember, there are all types of race participants. I take pride in being a BOTPer as I am a turtle and I will never win the Boston marathon. I do however think it would be really cool to qualify for it, and finish it one day, but I also know realistically there are amazing marathoners out there and I am just not one of them. I take pride in MY race now. I race against myself and that is enough of a race.

<u>November 13, 2015 – Facebook</u>

Distance: 5.13 miles

Time: 1:35:36

Pace: 18:37 min/mile

Today I am thankful for friends that will slow down their pace to walk with me; I finished the distance, just need to decrease the pace. Yay for negative splits!!! We did the training a day early. Much slower than I need it to be for the race. But basic math. 5 miles in 1.5 hours = 10 miles in 3 hours = 13.1 in a little less than 4 hours. Gotta get movin and groovin! :) So..... This may be a good time for you to laugh WITH ME... or at me. This weekend is a two-mile run. Next weekend is five miles. I was a week ahead of pace. Whoops.

Five miles. It turns out that I live exactly five miles away from my parents. I know that it is 3 songs in the car away, but I have never really given too much concern about the mileage, until training for a half marathon. It is amazing how creative you need to get. The best part of this post? No, not that I am Type A, not that I screwed up the mileage and ran 3 extra miles... that Carol trained with me. Carol – another sister from another mister. She could be my twin. We taught together for many years at the same brick and mortar school before moving to online education. So many students get us mixed up. Carol has an autoimmune disorder that has flipped her life upside down. Her faith and family see her through this nasty disease, and I know she will be kicking its ass for years to come! I will be right there next to her. (Love you, my sister!). What makes me so proud about this memory was the fact that while she was in the throes of this horrible disease, she had to slow down her running for me. Coaching me every step. Counting 1-100. Once we would get to 100 we would start over. It is amazing how you can do anything for 100 steps. We counted to 100 a lot on that training session, but it was worth it. I am sure looking back, that was the first time in my life I completed 5+ miles consecutively. Am I becoming a runner? I am still doing the intervals, but is this what a runner looks like?

November 16, 2015 – Facebook

Today I am thankful for others that believe in me, even when I cannot see it. I am finding during this running experience, I have the biggest cheerleaders, some that I would expect and others that are coming out of the woodworks! Some are passively kind ('Whatever you do, just don't stop'), and others that are in my face ('I will slap you with my phone if you talk negatively about yourself one more time during this race!') Both approaches are useful and needed. Thank you for my cheerleaders, or as this princess likes to call them - Fairy Godmothers!!!!

My self-doubt and insecurity continue to find a way to keep rearing their ugly face. It is remarkable. I was on this wonderful journey, and somehow, these anxieties kept creeping back in. Having strong people around you are so important. I was still judging myself by other's standards. I was not fast enough. I was still 326 pounds at this point. Goodness – how could I run this damn half marathon at 300+ pounds? There is no way I was going to finish this thing? I just knew I was going to be swept! There was just NO WAY I was going to finish! My knees were killing me, my feet were hurting me. With my background in athetic training, I was coming home and stretching, icing, using my stim unit – I was doing everything possible, but 326 pounds is 326 pounds. The force it puts on your body is undeniable.

When you cannot find the courage in yourself as those insecurities are creeping in, sometimes all it takes is a kind word from a friend, or encouragement from a stranger. It is funny, this is about the time that I started noticing all the people around my neighborhood that would be running. I would wave to them if I was in the car, still do to this day. A word of encouragement to a runner, walker, bicyclist goes a long way – you never know they might be doubting themselves. Be that positive word they are seeking to finish strong.

November 20, 2015 – Facebook

Distance: 5.19 miles

Time: 1:28:58

Pace: 17:09 min/mile

We went further this week and cut off 7 minutes!!! Today I am thankful for you. Carol, my coach. While you are more of a silent coach, I know you will not let me stop!

So, 7 minutes may not seem like a lot, but that is a little bit more than a minute per mile. That is huge! Especially when you know there are balloon ladies you need to be concerned about. In Disney races where they sweep, the last people to start, are a group of people that are lovingly known as the balloon ladies. They have this name as they have balloons tied to them, so you can see them coming. They keep a certain pace. If you are in front of them, you are technically okay, and should not be swept. If you are behind them, you are in jeop- ardy of being swept during the race. Typically, the pace is a 16-minute mile.

November 20, 2015 – Facebook

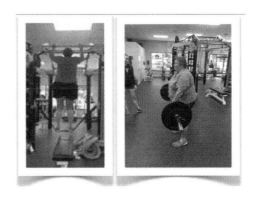

Pull-ups. My nemesis. 5 not enough. I will do 10, showing them who is boss. Mom is showing that age is just a number!

I hate pull ups. I HATE PULL UPS! This completely comes from elementary school PE. I remember Brentwood Elementary in Sarasota, FL in the 1980s... the dreaded Presidential Physical Fitness test. Why was I never sick on that day? UGH! All the boys could do so many pull ups. It felt like they could do over a hundred. It was probably closer to 10 or 20. Then the coaches would test the girls and maybe one or two girls could a handful of pull ups. I never was able to do one. My arms would be tighter than the knots in my stomach.

Here I am at 39, and my trainer tells me I am going to do pull ups? It takes me right back to that playground 30 years ago. I could still smell the wet grass, and the knots in my stomach returned. She placed a resistance band for me to step on. They gave way, so while I was pulling up, it was assisting, but I was still completing the motion. Talk about a confidence booster! I completed ten pull ups. TEN PULL UPS! This may not sound like a lot to many of you, but let me remind you, 326 pounds. Basic math... 326*10

pull-ups = 3260 pounds. Lots of weight lifted there!
I was not the only one making strides that day. I look over and my mom, is doing dead lifts. Wait a second. My mom – the woman was 65 years young at the time, has never so much as as lifted a weight bar in her life, and she is in beast mode! To say I am proud of her is an understatement! Mom and I were working out together. We were not running races together (yet…) but we were working out in the gym. Who starts deadlifts at 65? Fancy Nancy does – That's who!

November 23, 2015 – Facebook

7.3 miles go me!

Running has become my peaceful time. Many of the trainings by this point were my alone time. While some were with Carol and I still walked daily with Kelley (still do to this day!), my training runs were where I did my best thinking. I am sure that there is a peer-reviewed study that says there is an emotional/mental health benefit to running. I can tell you – there was a spiritual/emotional/mental connection for me personally. I had many conversations with God. I had many conversations with myself, and many times, I just found peace.
Mostly my long runs were on weekend mornings. I missed church. I missed Saturday morning breakfasts with family. This was my time by myself. No one was watching and it was okay as it was what I needed. Then there were the times that I would be training, and I would hear a horn honking, and it would be my parents cheering me on, slowing down and encouraging me to continue on! Letting me know that they would be ready with food for fuel when I was done… keep going – I had this. God knows I love those two. They are my rock.

November 26, 2015 - Facebook

Today I am thankful for my dad. Sometimes I forget how lucky I am that I get to hang with him all the time. Including this morning at the Turkey Trot!!!! Here's to some Doobie Brothers and Crosby Stills and Nash (but no Young. He ruined the group). Love you dad!!!

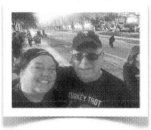

If we race on Thanksgiving, that is an extra piece of pie, right?

My dad is pretty cool. Bobby-T, as I lovingly call him, completed the Turkey Trot with me this year, as he did the year prior too. Knowing that I had the half marathon coming up, I wanted to run a race successfully with the intervals, and this was a great opportunity to practice. He let me run ahead and do so. My nieces and brother-in-law were at the finish line as they had already completed, and my sister walked with my dad. It may have just been a mile, it may have just been a fun run, but it did not matter, it was much more about my psyche than the physical run. Sometimes that is what the run is about that day – making sure your mind is right. For the record, many people will disagree with my music theory…. But I sure do love some "Southern Cross".

November 28, 2015 – Facebook

Distance: 6.70 miles

Time: 2:02:52

Pace: 18:20 min/mile

We did a little more than a half of a half!!!! The negative splits were on the downhill miles.

Half of a half! The weather was beautiful on that day! Lots of deer cheering us on. I was finding it easier to breathe. Was it the weather? Was it my body becoming it accustomed to the training? Was it both? I know it was not the weight loss, because there was none! To say there was a certain level of frustration is an understatement. UGH. How do you train for as long as I have been training, fueling your body for a race and still not losing any weight? This does not make sense.

December 5, 2015 - Facebook

Distance: 3.72 miles

Time: 1:01:24

Pace: 16:34 min/mile

Thinking outside of the box. What do you do when you are trying to run part of the race path for a training run, and then you remember that the sidewalk stops at MK and picks back up at Grand Floridian???? Take a boat of course! I wonder if they have this option during the race.... Either way - beautiful morning to be at Disney. I love when my run ends at my castle. With my soldier out front guarding.

Losing One Hundred Pounds

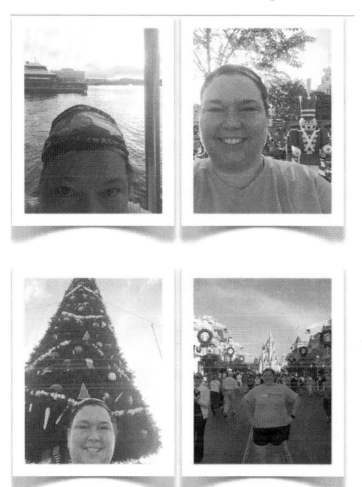

Clara Boyd

We go to Walt Disney World every December to spend time with friends that are visiting from New Jersey. Once again, friends that are like family…My dearest memories from years past include this group. This trip to Disney was different. I was on a mission. This was the last trip I would take there before the race. I needed to train and run as much of the race course without going to "Disney Jail". I don't know if there is really such a place, but I did not want to find out. The half marathon course starts just outside of EPCOT, travels down the highway to the Magic Kingdom, through the Magic Kingdom (including the castle), past The Grand Floridian, the Polynesian, Mile 10 of the race is an on ramp of a highway, through EPCOT, and finishes in the EPCOT parking lot. So, while I could not legally run the course, I figured I would run part of the course. My fears were calmed a bit. I needed this training. Mind over matter. Again.

December 11, 2015 - Facebook

Distance: 8.32 miles

Time: 2:32:55

Pace: 18:34 min/mile

No forest animal or Prince Charming on a horse will get me across the finish line, but training with one helluva fairy godmother will.

Carol. Again. She got me through this run. Cindy passed us on this run as did Carol's hus- band. The distance was improving, and I was staying on track. Trying to stay positive.
Proud of myself for the mileage but worried about the time. I was having nightmares of the balloon ladies and getting swept.

December 11, 2015

Funny thing happened on this Friday. While I was still weighing 326 pounds. (I really do hate my thyroid.) I am finally seeing a change in my body. At this point, my size 26 jeans are no longer fitting. They are falling off! I had to go buy new jeans. I might not have been in single digit jeans, but this is progress. Changes are happening.

Christmas 2015 - Facebook

Life is slowly getting back to normal. Dad is finally home, and mom is yelling at the foot-ball refs on the TV. Lol. Will go for a run in the morning. 9.5 miles is what I need to complete for the training. I may go to sleep right now to prepare.

Christmas 2015 was not the best for my family. Mom had a scheduled knee surgery right before Christmas, and dad had an accident on the day that mom was being discharged from the hospital resulting in both of them being laid up for weeks with leg injuries. I am continually reminded that life continues to happen no matter your plan. Many times, during this turbulence, I would pray the Serenity Prayer. I never understood it, until I really needed it in my life.

December 26, 2015 – Facebook

Distance: 9.56 miles

Time: 2:59:34

Pace: 18:46 min/mile

It was ugly but it is done. This is nowhere in track to keep pace for the Princess half but today was more mental than anything. It is done.

REPLY TO CAROL'S MOM - *Love you too Mamama. I could not have done it without Carol. She has been my therapy thru all of this. Xoxo*

POST ON A RUNNER'S BLOG - *This has been a crazy week for me - both of my parents are injured right now with leg injuries and so I have moved back in to be the primary caregiver. I have not trained in a week, nor slept well (the couch is now my bed until mid-January), nor have I really worried about my nutrition. I told my sister last night that I was going to withdraw from the PHM if I could not get out and train today (5-minute pity party). It was the worst run ever, but emotionally it was what I needed. Thank you to eve-ryone in this group, as I feel that we are all here to support each other! Reading your posts are what kept me putting one foot in front of the other today!*

Clara Boyd

REPLY TO A RUNNER ON A BLOG - Aimee - I had to take a look back at all the hard work I have done for this run, and I thought - I cannot give up. Life 'gets in the way', for lack of a better term. It was rough to get out there today. I do not want to get picked up by the busses, but as I trained today, all I could think was - any distance is better than not trying at all. Praying for you!

There is something to be said about getting up and getting back out there. Putting one foot in front of the other and just get moving – no matter how slow. The time of this run was horrible, but that did not matter. 9.56 miles was amazing. My sister and I were now the primary caregivers for my parents, who both needed a lot of medical attention. Mom just had major surgery, and dad was about to have major surgery. I was sleeping on their family room couch, as staying in their guest bedroom was too far away from the recliners they were sleeping in, if they needed something in the middle of the night, which was approximately every 2 hours. To say we were all sleep deprived was an understatement. But they are family. And that is what you do. I would not change a thing because I know they would do the same for me – and they have. That is life. That is love. That is family.

January 1, 2016 – Facebook

Shout out to my workday walking buddy Kelley! This is the first New Year's resolution I actually kept! How about another year of morning walks and gossip???

Did I really just keep a New Year's Resolution for an entire year?

Hell yeah, I did!

January 7, 2017 – Facebook

Happy moment of the day... Trainer at the gym told me that I inspire her to run! Here's a woman that I look up to every week for guidance and she is actually looking up to me as well! My heart is very happy! Also ran a sub 16-minute mile in the gym, I know I can do it! I'm going to finish this half marathon!

Kolbey is such an inspiration to me. She is 15 years younger than me, but then again, age is merely a number. If you have not learned this yet in this chapter with my mom doing dead-lifts at 65, you will understand it now. Kolbey was born when I was a freshman in high school. How can this girl have any influence on my life? She is the one that got me to do a pull up, ten of them to be exact. Right there that should tell you something! From one-on-one chats during workouts to motivational texts to keep me going, Kolbey has a heart of gold. She has become more than just a trainer, but a good friend. At this point you know what happens when someone becomes a friend, they become family, a sister! The fact that she told me that day that I inspired her to run, I was humbled. There are few times in my life that I have been truly humbled. This was one of them. With the stress that occurred with my family the past few weeks, to have Kolbey say these kind words, and then to run a sub 16-minute mile, my confidence was starting to increase.

January 17, 2016 – Facebook

"Energy and persistence conquer all things" Benjamin Franklin

As this race is getting closer - 5 weeks from right now - this is so true. I am proud of myself and everyone else that has the courage to have a goal, to be vulnerable enough to embrace your weaknesses to achieve this goal, and the strength to follow through.

January 21, 2016 – Facebook

A gentle reminder - the half marathon is ONE MONTH FROM TODAY!!!! No, I am not stressed at all! :) Actually, I am so excited. This is one journey I never thought I would take, but proud of it, no matter what the outcome!!!

I was starting to get very excited about the race and felt a moment of peace. It was the first time that I could see the fun in this journey. Before me was such a monumental goal that I never thought in my life I could achieve, and it was only a month away. I was going to achieve it!

January 26, 2016 – PHM

So, the race nightmares have officially started. I dreamt last night that I was at the Contemporary at the time the race started and I was begging for someone to drive me to EPCOT. The Disney reps told me they could not because Hillary Clinton was staying there and they were not allowed to leave. I am not staying at Contemporary and we all know I am so OCD that I will be the first one to the start of the race. Sigh.

Well, that sense of fun was short lived….

Many runners will tell you that there are nightmares that occur before races, and I certainly had my share of them. Missing the start of the race was a recurring one. I would wake up with night sweats, rapid heartbeat, and try to go back to sleep…all while praying that I would just survive the race.

January 28, 2016 – Facebook

Rowing, pulling ropes, flipping tires, just to name a few. All before 8:30. Then coming out to the car to hear EYE OF THE TIGER blasting. Yeah - it's going to be a great day!

Kolbey inspiring me again…being a Clemson Tiger? You KNOW *Eye of the Tiger* is my song! GO TIGERS!

January 28, 2016 – Facebook

How interesting I saw this post this today. Earlier this week, I had a conversation with a male friend who says that people treat him differently when he is at a lesser weight than he is now. Funny thing - I have never looked at him as overweight. But then I again - I see a kind human being; not their weight, their race, their religion. With that being said, I had a conversation with my trainer today about the fact that I am my own worst critic and how I analyze my physical attributes way too harshly. I guess others are their own worst critics as well.

We have been friends since middle school. Never have I seen him as an obese guy, skinny guy, lesser of a friend because of his size – I just see him as a friend, brother, and a person with the biggest, kindest heart ever. This study ("Obese women experience much more negative social stigma than previously thought, study finds") in the *Journal of Health Psychology* discusses the stigmatism associated with obese women, and the comments that people, including family and friends, make to them on a daily basis. The citation is at the end of the book, so if you are so inclined, please feel free to read the article. It is an interesting article but brings up a bigger concern.

Why do people feel they have the right to make comments? Throughout my life people – be it friends, family, acquaintances or complete strangers, felt they had the right to tell me about my weight, my size, and what was "best" for me to do. While they may have been saying this out of concern or love, it was not taken that way, and it was NOT OK. I always took these comments as if I was being treated differently, and added to my insecurities. I remember being younger and being told "You would be skinnier if you…", or "You would be prettier if you…". People don't recognize how emotionally damaging this is? These words I still hear to this day. I understand that this was a different time and that people "know better" now, but that doesn't make it right. I will admit, I was once one of those people, allowing my own insecurities to come through and giving advice to others on how to lose weight. I am truly sorry if I ever made you feel insecure, or less than amazing. YOU ARE AMAZING! Remember that always. No one has the right to use negative words, especially if you are not a model of perfect health. If you feel that you want to help someone with a weight problem, do it through modeling the behavior. Let me explain. Looking back, as an overweight child, I would have much rather had an adult model a healthy behavior for me than belittle me. I love that in my family we all participate in races, we all go to the gym, we model healthy behaviors. Do we always make the best choices? No, but we make a conscious effort. We are not perfect. We are human.

However, with this race, there was something happening. I was finding my confidence in the fact that I was about to complete a half marathon, something that a year ago I would have never imagined, and I was gaining confidence in myself. That confidence goes beyond the number of miles run!

February 2, 2016 – PHM

I found out my bib number!!!! I will not be in the last corral!!!! I am so exited - this is so real! I want to go run right now to train!!!!

I was not going to be in the last corral! This is important! Those balloon ladies were in the last corral! This gave me a buffer, if you will, as there were many people between me and the balloon ladies. Think of it as me getting a really big head start on the balloon ladies.

February 5, 2016 – Facebook

2 weeks! 2 weeks! Eeekkkk!

The old me – you know, the one that would have given up? Sat on the side of life? Made excuses? – I was not losing to her again, I will beat her. I could not go back. I refused to.

February 6, 2016 – Facebook

Tiger Lily is ready with 2 weeks to spare. The final long run is tomorrow. All that's left now is to get to Disney and enjoy the moment!!!! (The paper that you see in the final picture is the 'contract' my fashion designer - aka Alex- made me fill out for the 7-dollar charge to create my costume. What a little entrepreneur!)

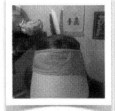 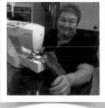 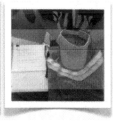

I was in full race mode at this point. Preparations were in full swing! My mom sewed the final touches on my race costume. My niece wrote a contract for "Grandma's Sewing Services". That was the best $7.00 I have ever spent on clothes!

February 7, 2016 – PHM

Distance: 12 miles

Time: 3:02:46

Pace: 15:19 min/mile

Last long run before the big day is done!!!!! I feel good about it :)

In 3 hours, I completed 12 miles. That is on average a 15-minute mile. I had confidence that I was going to complete this half marathon. That was also in a controlled environment. No other runners, on the treadmill, no turns, no Mile 10 ramp. Just me and the treadmill.

February 14, 2016 – Facebook

I have the best nieces! They got me a bag full of gummy bears for Valentine's Day - EXACTLY what I will eat during my race!!!!

I have the coolest nieces. I had figured out if I ate a few gummy bears every 4 miles, I would have enough carbohydrates to push through until the next 4-mile mark during the race. Now, any runner will tell you, you NEVER change anything on race day. This could have serious implications on your GI system, and you do not, I repeat – DO NOT want to use the port-o-potty if you do not need to. Thus, during my longer runs, anything beyond 4 miles, I would eat approximately 10 gummy bears. I remember praying that I would not choke on a gummy bear. That would be my luck – "Did Clara get swept because of her mile time? Did she fall and sprain an ankle? NO! She choked on a yellow gummy bear – not even the red one. The yellow one." Damn.

<u>February 17, 2016 – Facebook</u>

I get in the car and this song is on. What a flashback to high school! But as I packed the car to head to Orlando for my race, this is truly THE TIME TO REMEMBER! Just a quick trip to the Capitol to see some friends and remind them why I work for the most innovative educational company in the world, and then it is off to THE WORLD!

The song, *"This is the Time to Remember"* by Billy Joel takes me back to my high school days, as it was used for our senior year video. And how amazing of a song it is! – just so meaningful to many times during our lives.

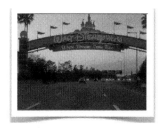

"Where Dreams Come True"

<u>February 20, 2016 – Facebook</u>

So, if you did not know, I am running a little race tomorrow. (And if you did not know, that means you blocked me about 10 months ago). But this journey started a long time before that.

About 9 years ago, one of the bravest princesses I know started fighting one helluva battle. As she battled with leukemia, I wanted to run the

Disney Princess Half Marathon. I thought of every excuse. I am too old, I am too out of shape, I don't have time, I am too big, you name it I found the excuse. And then I remembered her. If she could fight as hard as she was - I could run a measly 13.1 miles.

Fast forward 9 years, and I am about to run this race. Yes, it took me a while to get here, but I am here. I will not be the fastest out there. Hell - I may be the slowest. But I will be there, and that is all that matters to me.

I want to thank my Fairy Godmothers and Godfathers. My mom and dad have supported this crazy idea from the beginning. **Nancy and Robert.** *My sister that trained with me to be supportive; Valerie who made me run even on vacation (that won't be happening in a week); my nieces - the two best trainers/supporters I know - I hope I make you proud; and everyone else there are so many of you to name - I could not do this without the love and support you have shown. Carol, Cindy and Laura - my girls that were crazy enough to join me on this journey. What the heck are we thinking? Love you all!*

So tomorrow will be for the princesses that can't run for themselves, the princesses right beside me, in front of me and behind me. To the princesses that think they are too old (you know who you are, 50 is but a number), to the princesses who want to run but are too scared to try, to the princesses that think - I will be swept by the bus - it all starts with the first step.

Now – let's get this party started!!!

<u>February 21, 2016 – Facebook (VERY EARLY)</u>

Get up every one! It's race day!!!

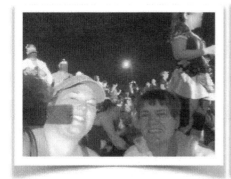
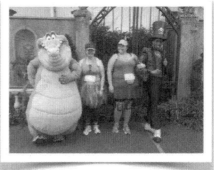
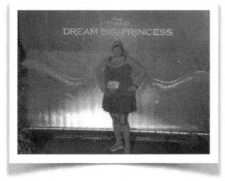

Carol and me (Top Left),

Louis, Laura, me, and Dr. Facilier from "The Princess and the Frog" (Top Right),

Me - Dreaming BIG! (Bottom)

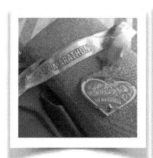
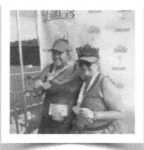

BLING BLING!!!

And 4 hours and 19 minutes later....

I did it! We finished complete back of the pack. As in last. But I did it.

February 23, 2016 – Facebook

Losing One Hundred Pounds

Many years ago, I wanted to run a half marathon. I figured it would be a cool thing to accomplish. But how could I do it? I was overweight, out of shape, and did not have the time. When I would try to run, I would be out of breath before I made it fifty yards!

So many times, people would offer me encouragement and support to start this journey, but I would still find excuses... until I realized I was going to be 40. I have done a lot in my life that I am proud of in the past 39 years, but there was one thing that was in the back of my mind... I did not complete a half marathon.

There was a specific half that I had my eye on.... The 2016 Disney Princess Half Marathon on February 21st. I had to sign up in June of 2015 – it was all a fantasy and exciting, until you pay a lot of money to run. And then you get nervous and anxious at the same time and realize – I cannot fail.

In March of 2015, I started training. Actually, I started training to train. Meaning – I had to get in shape to even start the real training for the race. I bought a few apps for my phone, new shoes, new workout clothes; I was ready for anything! I utilized the Jeff Gallo- way method; running/walking intervals. For those that do not know what that means, you run for a specific amount of time, and then walk for a specific amount of time. I found that 40/40 intervals fit me best. So, I would run for 40 seconds, and then walk for 40 seconds. I trained like this until October, when the official Disney training started.

I trained with family members, friends, on vacation, on business trips, I made sure that I never missed a training. My plantar fasciitis would show its ugliness on the longer runs, which soon became walks. I knew that I needed to have a 16-minute mile or quicker to not get swept. See, the half marathon runs from EPCOT to Magic Kingdom and then back to EPCOT. There are highways, and exit ramps, bridges, and tunnels. In all fairness, Disney needs to move traffic through all of these areas, thus, if you do not keep up this pace, they will sweep you to make sure they can open back up the roads in a timely manner. If you ask anyone that has spoken to me since October 2015, somewhere in there I mentioned the 16 min mile or the balloon ladies. Ahhhhhhh – the balloon ladies, these women volunteer to walk a 16 min mile pace, and they are the very last runners to start the race. If you are behind them at certain parts of the race, you will be swept from the race, put on the "Parade Bus", and then sent to the finish line. They have balloons tied to their race outfits so that you can gage where you are in comparison, hence their name. I would come to find out that they are quite lovely ladies.

The plantar fasciitis really started becoming a hindrance with my running, as well as everyday life. I have put away my flip flops, heels, any shoe that did not have the word sneaker in it. My orthotic arch supports, heel cups, and ibuprofen have been my lifesavers for a few months now. I decided I needed to contact my orthopedic doctor and prayed to get an appointment the week after the race. His PA was able to see me approximately 1 month prior to the race. Long story short, I have a fracture in my left foot, as well as plantar fasciitis so bad that I will be having surgery in May. At no point did this deter me. I was not going to miss the race – pain is temporary, and I worked too hard (yes – I am stubborn)

The time comes to travel to the race. I drove to Orlando on Wednesday in preparation for the Race Expo that opened on Thursday morning. If you have never been to one, I highly recommend going to one – the people watching is unbelievable! I have mixed emotions about the expo. There are many wonderful exhibitors and runners alike. Great information to learn, and products too! I saw Jeff Galloway again, and spoke about running the hills of Tallahassee, something he has done a few times.

However, there are a few bad apples that can spoil the bunch. I was there, or should I say – I survived the expo. There were people fighting verbally and physically over jackets and wine glasses. I witnessed both, and it just made me sad. At what point have we become so ravenous over an object? Have we forgotten what the weekend was all about? And then I found out… many of the people in the expo were not runners, but people that planned on selling the merchandise online. We *were not even out of the expo before there were reports of items for sale online. Completely sad to see. But my main focus of the week was Sunday morning.*

So, after a few days of carb loading, and relaxing by the pool, it was time for the race!

Disney does a race day like no one else! While this was my first half marathon, it was certainly not my first rodeo. I have done local races which are great, and always for a great cause, but the money that Disney puts into every detail – wow. From the moment we walked off the bus at EPCOT, you could feel the excitement in the air. To say I was nervous was an understatement, but the excitement was outweighed any nerves.

After a 20-minute walk to the corrals (yes – 20 minutes) I waited with 24,000 of my closest friends getting ready for the run of my life. After the national anthem from Miss America, some fireworks, and a few prayers sent above, it was my time to go!

As much as I wanted to run, I knew I needed to save my energy, and so speed walking it was! I set my eyes on another runner and kept pace with them. Within 2 miles, my friend caught up to me and we were ready to walk the rest of the way in stride.

One foot in front of the other. That is how we would make it. Some things you find out during 13.1 miles: humility, strength, perseverance. Around mile 8 we hit a low. We had some choices to make and we decided to dig deep. When I was doubting myself, Laura was there to push me. When she was down, I did the same for her. About this time, the balloon ladies caught up with us. Through my nervousness, I asked them loudly if they were the legitimate balloon ladies. If by some chance they read this, I want them to know – I admire you, and did not mean to yell – I was speaking loudly through fear and nerves. I was watching them disappear into the distance. At this point, I came to the realization that I was going to be swept. I made peace with it. What I could not make peace with was getting the medal. In my opinion and in my heart – I did not deserve a medal stating that I completed a half marathon if I did not earn it. (Disney still gives the runners who were

Clara Boyd

*swept the medal. I am not degrading their efforts, and I could quite possibly be in their shoes – There is an emotion affiliated with crossing the finish line after 13.1 miles that you cannot explain) And then I got a text. A dear friend of mine who was also running the race had finished with grace. A text from her popped up on my watch. "When your legs get tired...Run with you HEART!!" and that is what I did. We started to speed up our pace. And then we saw the waving flags. Over a megaphone a race official started saying that we had one minute to get past him so that we did not get swept. We were about 50 yards away from him. There was no way.... but my perseverance was greater than the negative thoughts in my head. We **ran. Hard.** We did not look back.*

Up the mile 10 ramp we started to go. I was so focused on getting up the ramp, I could not hear anything going on, or lack thereof. About half way up the ramp, I turned around to see the 6000 (yes – 6000) people behind me... and no one was there. At that very moment I realized – we did not get swept! Could it be that I may actually finish this? I still had an entire 5K ahead of me. Within the last 3 miles, Laura and I met up with a lovely lady from Tennessee named Mary Leigh. We were all three going to finish this race. With every step we encouraged each other. While the medics on bikes circled us like sharks, we kept moving forward.

When we reached the edge of EPCOT, I finally felt that we would not be swept. I cried. An ugly cry. But I kept moving forward. The volunteers cheered us on (Major shout out to all of the volunteers with the race – they are amazing people and deserve a round of applause) The tourists in EPCOT cheered us on. The cast members cheered us on. The gospel choir cheered us on – actually, started walking with us in support. As we turned the corner to finish the race, another runner slowed down and ultimately was the last to finish. I finished the race hand in hand with one of my best friends, we crossed the line with my family and friend cheering us on.

It has been 24 hours since the race. Many people have told me I would catch the bug and be ready to sign up for my next half marathon. I have not caught that bug, and probably won't. But 5Ks sound amazing! In fact, I will be signing up for many more in the future…

I cannot thank my family and friends for all the encouragement and support over the past year. I would not have been able to complete this journey without each and every one of them.

I am so grateful – not only to my friends and family, but to myself. I allowed myself to be vulnerable; to be hurt; to feel defeated; to find peace; to find strength; to persevere through trials; to be successful. I have accomplished a goal that was out of reach for so long – and now it is a box checked on my bucket list. BIG Girls Rule – and we ruled it for 13.1 miles.

LETTING GO OF THE WEIGHT

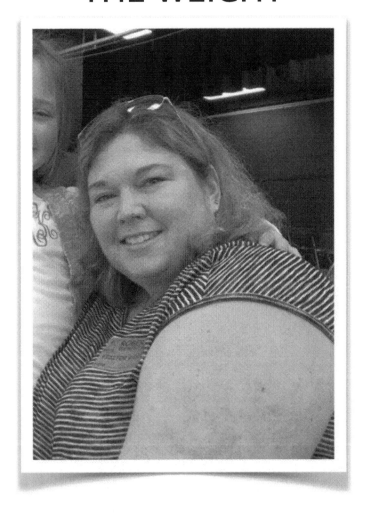

The Half Marathon ticker-tape celebration is long over, and life has gotten back to normal. Work, family, stressors, and 326 pounds. During the race, I lost 3 pounds, however, I also ran the race with a fractured left foot, and an injured left plantar fascia. I had surgery on the plantar fascia, and while the surgery went great, an infection set in afterwards. Thus, I could not exercise afterwards. My 40th Birthday I woke up in Aruba, depressed, but wanted to put on a smile for family. Things had to change, or I was not going to see 41...

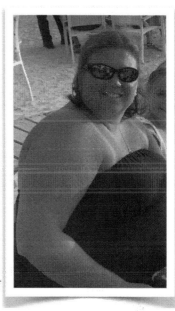

Aruba, July 13, 2016
Weight - 326 pounds
Fake smile, as I was not happy with myself

January 30, 2017 - Facebook

It has been a while since I have written, I have been "under construction". I thought about whether to even write this blog, and many friends told me not to, as it is no one's business, and it is true – my journey really is no one's business other than my own. I do not write this for the attention, I do not write this for the pat on the back. I am writing this, because maybe I can help someone out there. As they say –

Clara Boyd

if one person reading this is inspired or educated, then it is worth it! So – if you do not want to read the story of my weight journey, please feel free to close this, and continue to read about political posts, or look at someone's pictures of their dinner.

OK – here we go. This is ME.

My name is Clara, and I am addicted to food. To say it is freeing, and a little cheesy, but it is true. I love food – I sound like a commercial with Oprah in it – but I am being real. I enjoy making food, I enjoy the social aspect that it brings, I enjoy the taste – I just don't enjoy the cleaning dishes.

I have always been the biggest of all of my friends. In high school, I was 6 feet tall, weighed 199 pounds, I was a size 12/14, and I thought I was disgustingly obese. I look at pictures of myself back then and think – I would give anything to look like that again. I know a lot of people who wish they could look like they did at 17. I just wish I could go back to my 17-year-old self and tell her to own it! Screw what all of the magazines said. She was sexy, she was smart, and had a lot to offer people. I am so thankful that this generation coming up is living in a time where the media is recognizing its influence, and the fact that they can make a positive change in body image.

My professional career had allowed me to justify making poor nutritional choices. Being an athletic trainer, I have eaten more hot dogs out of hydrocollators, drive-thru meals, concession stand dinners, team meals at midnight, you name it – I have the excuses. This, plus hypothyroidism and PCOS has led me to weighing 326 pounds. Saying that makes my stomach turn. I never imagined tipping the scales at 320, but I did. But do you think that made me take control – nope. Finding out that I was pre-diabetic, on 2 blood pres- sure medicines, and going down a path that would end in cardiac problems…would that make me take control? Nope. Do you know what did? Turning 40.

Let's take a step back. Many people have addictions. Drugs, smoking, other lifestyle choices that can be addicting – whatever it is. I am not belittling any of them. Everyone is on their own journey. I believe it was Al Roker that said, and I paraphrase, that eating is the only addiction that you have to continue to have in your life. You can go without alcohol, drugs, etc., but you still have to eat food. Knowing this addiction is something that I will deal with every day for the rest of my life is humbling and hard. Someone very dear to me asked me a few months ago – why don't you just cut back on what you are eating? I wish it was that easy. I wish I could just "put down the sandwich" and BAM – I would lose 5 pounds. And while I am on that subject – losing weight is not the same for everyone. Some that need to lose 5-10 pounds to fit into their bikini is a heck of a lot different from a morbidly obese person that needs to lose 50+ pounds to save their life. I respect anyone that is trying to lose weight, even 5-10 pounds, but that is comparing apples to oranges (look at that – a food comparison…. sigh).

To say I have tried every diet is an understatement. If it is out there, I have tried it. I even sold some of them! I went to a meeting about bariatric surgery – I was denied by my insurance. Looking back now, I am happy I was. But the response I got when I questioned why it would not be covered…. It is not cost efficient for them. (Hmmmm – OK – so the multiple medications I am on, and potential diseases and the costs of all of that is cost efficient…OK) Let me also say – there is not a 'one size fits all' when it comes to dieting. What may work for some, will not work for others. Twice in my life, I bought into 2 very well-known dieting plans. One included a lot of vitamins and a 21-day cleanse, and the other included daily shakes. I have dear friends that these products are working for. Both even worked for me in the sense of my blood work. I was taking a pre-diabetic level A1C and moving back into a normal range. What was not moving in the right direction was my weight. I was justifying that if my blood work looked good, it didn't matter what was on the scale.

At this point, you may be thinking – well, hello – how about adding in exercise. I have paid for a personal trainer for the past 6+ years. I had been working out long before then. I was working out, but not working on me. I was going through the motions. It is hard to push through and work harder when you are trying to fit onto the machines, or there is someone next to you on a treadmill who is running, while texting, watching the television, not breathing hard, and barely breaking a sweat…and there I am holding on praying to not walk sideways off the treadmill. Remember – I am the klutz that broke my foot on an elliptical in college. Yes, I did – that story is for another time.

Before turning 40, I wanted to complete a half marathon. I talk about that a lot in my earlier posts. You can read the details there. I trained for approximately 1 year for the race. I changed my eating habits, increased my exercise obviously, and in the entire process, I lost 3 pounds. THREE WHOPPING POUNDS! Wow! That is impressive – you have to try really hard to only lose 3 pounds after running hundreds of miles (that is also due to the thyroid and PCOS). So, I walk/ran a half marathon at 323 pounds. To say that my knees/hips/ankles were not in pain is ridiculous. I ended up needing foot surgery post-race, so I found those 3 pounds again really quick. So, on my 40th birthday, I was right back up to the 326 pounds.

With all of that said, I was proud of myself and all of my accomplishments. But do you know what was bothering me the most? The fear that I had when I was going to get on a plane. In my lifetime, I have done a lot for others. I believe in giving to others, helping others out. I still believe that; but with my 40th birthday coming up, I decided to start living for myself as well. I was going to take the trip, I was going to run the race, I was going to go and do…. I was ready to live for me. But getting on the plane and sitting in a plane seat is one of the biggest stressors in my life. As frustrating as it is that you may have to sit next to a large person on a plane, do you know what is going through their mind?

Let me take you through it –

<u>Step 1 – Buying the plane ticket….</u> OK, let me find a seat that possibly no one else will sit next to me; that way if I need to put the armrest up, no one will say anything to me. If the plane is packed, God please let there be an aisle seat so I can lean into the aisle the entire time (and pray that no one needs to get up), or a window seat so I can lean into the wall the entire time and pray that I do not need to get up.

Step 2 – Get to the airport. *Dear God, please let me get on the plane early, speak to the flight attendant quietly and ask for a seat belt extender – hoping there is one available, not the one they will use for the demonstration and will have to hand to you in front of a full plane; and then watch you to ensure you have it all clicked prior to takeoff. (And yes, that has happened to me)*

Step 3 – Get to the seat, hopefully with a seat belt extender in hand, click it onto the smaller seat belt, sit down, and quickly put the armrest up, so that expectation is there; praying that when the person sits next to you, they do not choose to put down the arm rest. Only one time in my flying days did someone give me a dirty look, and slam the armrest down, leaving one heck of a bruise on my hip. Trust me – I am not excited about the fact that my hips are invading in your armrest area. I am embarrassed and praying for the entire flight that you do not make a rude comment or tell the flight attendant that I am in your space.

Step 4- Survive the flight without eating the snack – as you are completely judged with every bite you eat, hold your drink of water, because you cannot fit in the seat with the tray down all of the way, and keep your arms crossed at all times, praying that the pain you are feeling from leaning into the aisle or the window the entire time will go away before you get on the next leg of your flight.

THAT is what the large person next to you is thinking on every flight. Life is going to happen, I am going to take that trip, and I may be sitting next to you on a flight. So, if I am – I am sorry.

Moving forward, I had a few scares this year including a genetic testing that showed an increase in my chances of various cancers including breast, skin, ovarian, colon, and thyroid. There is that word again – thyroid. In the midst of all of this, my annual ultrasound on my thyroid showed new masses, and the previous ones had grown in size. Lovely. Here I am, officially 40, officially larger than offensive linemen on football teams, increased chance of various cancers, and now having a biopsy done for thyroid cancer. It is pretty amazing the thoughts that go through your head as you are wide awake, lying on a table, head completely extended back, and being told not to move as a doctor has a needle the size of a pen in your neck. I needed to change my life. Starting with my weight. My chance of some of these cancers was increased even more because of my size. Shopping at a regular store? Out of the question. I am shopping online as living in a smaller town – there are no stores other than one particular superstore that has clothes large enough for you. And size 24 clothes were getting tight, real tight. As in – I would put on shorts with a zipper and a button, pray that the button did not pop, and that the red indentation in my skin around my waist would be gone by morning time the next morning. If I was going to live life to the fullest it started on that table. (Note: The biopsy showed all benign masses. Here's to them staying that way!)

*I decided to take another look at the bariatric center here in town. Not so much for the surgery, but for other options. I am a health educator, I have the knowledge – I just did not have the willpower. It is much more than just having the knowledge. Remember earlier in this post, I said that there is not a 'one size fits all' model with dieting. I am not endorsing this product, or this process; all I am saying is that this worked for me. The local hospital here has a program where the patients are put on Optifast shakes. I know what you are thinking – great – another option that is a quick fix and does not work as I will gain the weight right back. You may be right, but lord knows I hope to prove you wrong. Out of love and concern I have had dear friends that have questioned this process; not to be negative, but out of fear it is another failed attempt. Let me tell you why it won't fail. I am not going to let it. **I can't let it**.*

For the past 11.5 weeks, I have not eaten food. That's right – no Thanksgiving, no Christmas, no New Year's celebration. I was there for all of them, but I celebrated with everyone while they ate, and I did not. I have been on the Optifast program. This entails consuming 5 of their products daily. They have all of the nutrients you need to maintain daily functions, while being severely low in calories. To start out with, it is 5 shakes daily. My saving grace is that it is made by Nestle. So, while there is no bunny on the front of the package, I feel like I am drinking chocolate milk. You consume one every 3 hours, as well as at least 64 ounces of water throughout the day. I have always been a fan of water, so that second part was not hard. The shakes, well – that is another story. After 11.5 weeks, I never want to see chocolate shakes again. Ever. Prior to even starting the process, you get a full workup – stem to stern. A weight management doctor completes a full workup including physical, EKG, and blood work; a mental evaluation and physical history. After speaking with this physician, who is a well-educated Aussie who loves hugs, she advised me that a program as such would work well for me. With my medical history and fight- ing for so long to take control of this addiction, I need a strong intense program such as this one. And she was right.

The first day – God bless anyone I came in contact with that day. It was horrible. I was starting my official withdraw. I followed the plan perfectly, I was hungry – but I did not budge. I was not going to let this addiction beat me. By the end of the day I was hungry, exhausted, and just wanted to go to bed. When I got home, I needed to take in the garbage cans. As I was walking towards the garage with the garbage cans, the garage light had the audacity to turn off! That was the straw that broke the camel's back. I sat in my driveway and just cried. It was dark, no one could see me, so I let the tears flow. How did I let myself become 40, weigh 326 pounds, on the verge of some major medical problems, feel- ing completely lost and hopeless? … and my stomach is growling. I was so pissed at myself and allowed myself to have my pity party. For five minutes. It was cold and dark. Literally. But in Florida those mosquitoes will find you no matter the weather – so time to go inside, put on my big girl pants and deal with this head on. And I did. Every Monday I went to my weigh in, saw the doctor, got blood drawn, go to my group therapy to talk about the emotional challenges of food and weight issues, and then I would pick up my product and start another week of challenges. I have not cheated on this process not once. There are a few extrinsic factors…#1 – there is a chance of pancreatitis. I do not know how bad that hurts, and I do not want to find out. It is also life threatening. So, I figured - not taking the chance. #2 – this is expensive. Remember how I said that insurance would not pay for the bariatric surgery, where they would cut out my stomach? Well, they would not pay for this either. So, for the cost of a very nice trip to an exotic

Clara Boyd

Carib- bean Island for a week including travel and all other amenities, I am paying for this process. Just in case you forgot – I am a teacher – so this amount of money is huge to me. I cannot just throw this money around like it is nothing – it is an investment.

Each week, I continued to lose weight – sometimes 6-7 pounds, sometimes 1 pound. I am determined to beat this. I have walked daily with a friend, and gotten my butt kicked CrossFit style by my trainer on a regular basis. In 12 weeks, it is estimated to lose 50 pounds. Yesterday, I weighed in for my week 11. I have officially lost 51 pounds. It would be a Hallmark movie if I cried when I saw the number 269. But I didn't. I celebrated this milestone, got off the scale, and went to my doctor's appointment, including the EKG that you earn at the 50-pound mark, and then onto group therapy. It is interesting as there are people in there just starting this journey and hearing their fears and knowing those were my same fears 11 short weeks ago. And then I remember – this is real. I have lost more than 50 pounds. I am beating this addiction.

It is funny – there are some weeks, I cannot see a difference. I still see that fat woman praying to fit into the airplane seat. And then I look at my closet…. there are not a lot of clothes in there anymore. See, there is a group of us – 3 of us to be exact – that are trying to lose weight. One is counting calories and exercising, while another one is on the program with me. We are all being successful. We are sharing clothes, and then once they do not fit any of us, they are off to get donated. I will keep their names private, and respectfully hope you would do the same if you know who they are, as this is my story, and I want them to be able to tell theirs when they are ready if they decide to do so. Point being, we all share the same need – to lose a large amount of weight, but we are all on our own journey. I could not do it without these two beautiful amazing women in my life. Love you, ladies!

Right around the time that I had my biopsy done, the fall television shows were starting and there was one I was really interested in…. "This Is Us". I can honestly say that how they are portraying the weight struggles with Kate are pretty accurate in my case. (Minus the ease of getting the weight loss surgery done). There are people in your life that love you no matter your size. There are people who will judge you because of your size. But you are living in your skin and you know the pain and the struggle daily that goes along with being morbidly obese. My hat is off to the actress portraying Kate and thank her for showing the real struggles that go along with being obese. Now if I could find my Toby.... But that is for another post.

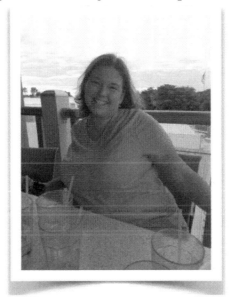

Above is a picture of me taken a few weeks back. At that point, I weighed 277. I had lost 43 pounds at that point and saw some friends and family I had not seen in years. Some had not seen me any larger than I was then, while others had seen me at a larger size, and knew the hard work I was putting into beat this addiction.

This is an addiction I will live with the rest of my life. I will be "under construction" and battle food every day. But I know that I will win this battle. Next Monday night, I will eat food again for the first time in 12 weeks – 4 oz of lean meat, and 1 cup of vegetables. I will gradually increase the amount of food and decrease the amount of Optifast product. To say I am scared is an understatement. The thought of food sounds great, but I am worried that the old habits will creep back in. You know the ones – walking by and grabbing a handful of crackers,

Clara Boyd

or coming home hungry and eating everything in sight, eating a huge bowl of ice cream while watching a movie, or just flat-out binging. This is a great time to talk about my support system. There are people in my life, that I cannot thank enough for various reasons, but there are people who have made this part of my journey possible. Some are local and see me daily, and some I have not seen since I started this but will see soon in February! The daily calls, the Monday morning texts asking how my weigh in went, the hugs, the positivity. You know who you are, as I did not share this journey with everyone. (I know – loud mouth me, actually kept something kind of quiet) Thank you. I love each and every one of you. I still need your support and your love. Going through this journey with all of you makes it easier on me and holds me accountable!

With all of that being said, I know we are all on our own journeys, and at different points in those journeys. I pray for all of you to attain your goals on your journey, whatever they are. I pray that you find your happiness.

This is ME, the skinnier version. All of my love – Clara

So, this is a great place to take a breather and explain how Optifast works. The program that I was involved in consisted of 5 nutritional products per day for 12 weeks. These products are shakes, soups, and bars that are high in protein, and low in calories. They are distributed by the medical facility that is affiliated with Optifast, and cannot be purchased righteously by a third party. After you have completed the initial 12-week phase, there is a transition phase for 4 weeks in which you begin to incorporate food back into your diet while supplementing with the products. After you have completed the intermediate phase, you begin what is called maintenance phase, which is ultimately your new lifestyle choices.

The Optifast Program does not just consist of the shakes, but regular doctor visits, the group therapy, and nutritionist visits. This is a yearlong commitment to the program, but in reality a lifetime commitment to your health. Specific group conversations therapy are confidential, however the topics included lifestyle habits such as stress eating, social aspects, celebrations around food, how to deal with eating on vacation, family and friend influences, and eating habits. Once the transition phase to food is incorporated back into your diet, the nutritionist appointments were integrated. She worked closely with me to ensure every calorie I was taking in had a purpose. I was learning to eat to live, not live to eat. Achieving maintenance means food was fully incorporated back into my diet, but I would continue to see the bariatric doctor once per month to ensure I stayed on track. I have the option to con- tinue this until I reach my weight goal and beyond, which for accountability purposes I plan to do.

February 6, 2017 – Facebook

Best first meal ever. 4 oz of fish. 1 cup of broccoli. Thank you, Logan. You did an amazing job! You hold a special place in all the Boyd's hearts!

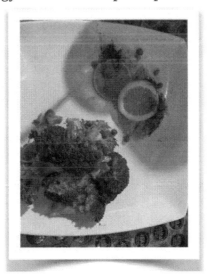

February 13, 2017 – Facebook

I have been thinking about this post now since I wrote the last one. First and foremost – many have reached out to me since I wrote. I appreciate every single person that reached out. Some publicly; some privately. Some for support, and some sharing their painful journey

Clara Boyd

that runs parallel to mine. I am grateful for all that are following this journey, for whatever your reason may be.

With that being said, this journey continues on…

I was driving in my car the other day, and on satellite radio is a comedian James Gregory doing a bit about the telephone. It was an older bit – talking about call waiting, caller ID, etc. He talked about how when he was younger, people would fight over who had to get up and get the phone because the phone was seen as an interruption to the day. The family would be on the porch (imagine Mayberry…) and RRRRRING! The family focus was disrupted. He then moved on to say that this day and age (maybe 20 years ago) that the problem was that life was interrupting the phone calls. People were more worried about what was going on other places and were too busy to take time to breathe and appreciate what was right in front of them. What would this comedian think of today's society?

One week ago tonight, I added food back into my journey. Now this part of the journey is big time baby steps. Last week I enjoyed 4 oz of meat and a cup of vegetables for dinner. That, accompanied by 4 of the Optifast products were my nutrition for the day. Being that my first meal was at the end of the day, last Monday was filled with anticipation. A local restaurant, who I consider the owners our friends, asked to cook our first meal. I was so excited and nervous at the same time. They took into consideration our limitations nutritionally and did an excellent job preparing a meal that they would not typically serve. (Broiled grouper and steamed broccoli) He plated the food beautifully – on a smaller plate. Remind me to talk to you about the plate size later….

As I sat there, excited like a kid on Christmas morning, not knowing which present to open up first – the broccoli or the grouper, I said a prayer of thanks – I was appreciative for that moment. I wanted to take everything in. The sight of the food, the smell of the food – and mostly the taste of the food. Needless to say, the grouper was amazing, the broccoli was perfectly al dente. Both flavored with lemons and spices. I enjoyed each bite, allowing the blend of flavors in the food to join together and create an amazing meal. What an experience! My love of food was back – but in a much different way. I loved appreciating the food to nourish my body. I appreciated the efforts put into making it for me. I appreciated the atmosphere. I appreciated the small plate. Wait – what??? 4 ounces of grouper and 1 cup of broccoli does not fill up a typical plate – but it surely filled my stomach, and my soul. I have heard this trick for years now – since I was in my Nutrition classes back at Clemson - A smaller plate tricks your mind into it believing you are eating more. (side note – the nutrition class was in the dairy building – the same one that the Clemson ice cream store was in…. every Tuesday and Thursday, we would walk into nutrition class with milkshakes… Hmmmm)

Well, thank goodness my parents have smaller plates at their home – who knew we would all be using them so fast! The next couple days included experimenting in the kitchen. Some nights were really yummy – some nights… well…. let's just say egg substitute and a cup of chopped onions and mushrooms do not cook together that well. I have once again found my love of being in the kitchen. Not just going through the motions; but really loving the act of cooking again. Thinking about which spices would enhance flavors of various proteins, which vegetables would complement the protein. How would I eat spinach without sautéing it in EVOO???…. which it can be done! A major shout out to my brother-in-law for steaming bags of spinach last night instead of sautéing it!

This brings me to my next thought – making cooking a family experience again. When did we stop enjoying this process as a group? If you know me, you know I love to cook for others, just ask anyone that would come to my apartment for egg sandwiches or chicken piccata in college – but that is another story for another time. More than cooking FOR friends and family, I enjoy cooking WITH friends and family. Together – creating a meal – such a great time of fellowship. One of my niece's favorite things to eat is meatloaf. Do you know why? Her first memory of meatloaf is when she pulled her stepladder over to the kitchen counter, and helped my mom mix all of the ingredients in the bowl, and then shape the meatloaf in the pan. She was so proud of her creation, she ate it! It was a break away from the chicken nuggets and Mac-n-cheese that children lean towards. I joke that they were not just making meatloaf, they were making memories. WOW – what an experience.

Too many of us are just going through the motions in life and missing the experiences. How many times have you cooked dinner, and eaten it all while thinking of other things going on in life – trying to get homework done, laundry folded, whatever it is – not truly enjoying the experience? Better yet, how many times have you driven through a fast food place or stayed in your car in the TO GO parking space, while someone else had your food waiting for you – even the plastic forks and knives, as you are too busy with other parts of life to make dinner. Trust me – I am not judging you; been there, done that, and probably was behind you in the Chick-fil-a line.

Sadly, this morning, while I was waiting to check in for my weigh in, the patient in front of me decided to quit the program. My heart is truly hurting for her tonight. Like I said in the last post, there is not one specific program that will work for everyone. She was not ready to take this journey. We had spoken in the past how she was too busy. As I watched her walk out of the waiting room, all I could think about was the satellite radio bit I heard. Are we too busy that we are allowing experiences to pass us by?

A new experience for me tonight on this journey. Today, along with my 4 oz of protein and a cup of vegetables, I added a small piece of fruit. You would have thought I was told I won the golden ticket! I was so proud to go to the grocery store and purchase fresh fruit. The choices were abundant. I was so excited – what would I add to nourish my body? So tonight – after my 4 oz of a sirloin burger with mushrooms and green beans, I enjoyed the sweetest and juiciest nectarine.

And for those that are wondering, I lost 4.5 pounds this week to total 58 pounds. More importantly, I was taken off Metformin – the final medicine I could be taken off of. (I will forever be on thyroid meds – no amount of weight loss can change that) Metformin, for those that do not know, is used for diabetic and pre-diabetic patients that controls blood sugar levels. Due to my weight loss and healthy lifestyle choices,

I was getting dizzy spells being on my prescription meds. A few weeks back I was taken off my blood pressure meds, and today, my pre-diabetes meds. This experience validates the past 14 weeks of hard work.

So, while I may not have a front porch like Mayberry, and my work life may be for one of the most innovative technology companies, I am making a commitment to enjoy more experiences... the big experiences!

All of my love ~ Clara

February 13, 2017 – Private Thoughts

Had an interesting situation happen today... I was cat called by the construction workers today outside of the gym as I walked out. That was a 'first' I was not ready for. What are you supposed to do - Smile? Wave? Ignore them?

I was walking out of the gym in my tank top and leggings. Apparently, my legs are getting pretty defined; defined enough that it was worth a whistle. Let me just say - I am not a pushover. I work hard professionally. If something needs to be fixed at my house, I will roll up my sleeves and fix it. But there is something to be said for when a man notices you. (And by the way men - cat calling is never going to make a lady change her plans - she will not come over and talk to you)

I have walked out of that specific gym door multiple times per week for 3+ years now. I have walked out of many gym doors for many years. No cat calls. Has my physique changed that much, or is it more how I carry my physique? I admit - I am starting to walk a little taller, a little more confident, and starting to be okay with my body.

And a stranger noticing my hard work every so often - for this gal at least - a confidence booster.

All my love ~ Clara

I do not believe in degrading anyone at any time. However, a little positive affirmation, letting someone know they look good is not a bad thing. I remember this day. The comments made were not degrading in anyway. If I am driving by you, and you are walking/running, etc., I will honk, wave, cheer you on – I believe in you, and support you in your efforts. By no means am I supporting degrading someone. I believe in lifting them up. (Side note – I would NEVER condone cat calling as a way to gain attention. It is degrading to anyone – men and women alike! While the comments made that day toward me were not depreciating, I know many times they are, and that should not be tolerated. I was just shocked that someone was noticing ME!)

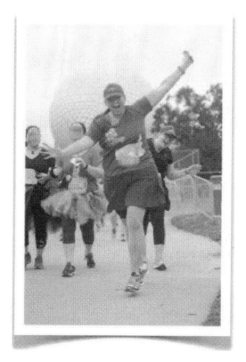

My Favorite PHOTOBOMB Ever!!!!

February 24, 2017 - Facebook

One of my favorite race pictures ever – me, EPCOT, and Laura peeking from behind me. The joy of racing at Disney with friends – one of my favorite things in life! We are pretty princesses for sure!

LETTING GO OF CONTROL

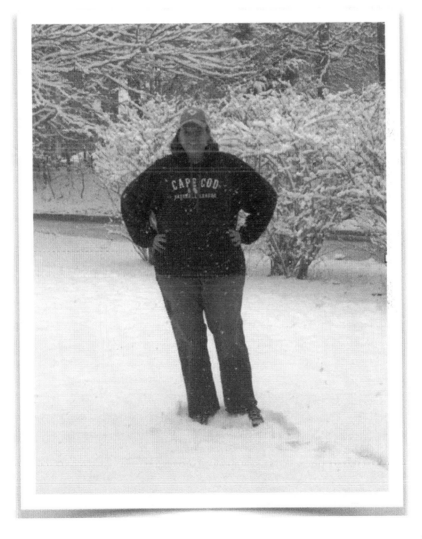

Clara Boyd

February 28, 2017 - Private Thoughts

I am so filled with emotions I do not know where to even start. Let's start with the positive – I ran a 5K... Three of them last week to be exact. See, there comes a point of time in your life when you realize your friends and family are the most important thing - and creating experiences with them is what matters in life. So, last week a group of us from all over the east coast met up to do a race at Disney. A Princess race if you will.... One of the girls - who is amazingly fit said that we should do a 5K every full day we were there. So, we did! It was a really positive experience knowing that I could complete them. And let's get something else out of the way - when I say I ran a 5K, I should clarify that and say that I completed the 5K. I normally do the Jeff Galloway method of walk-run-walk. With that being said - my running in the official 5K consisted of every time we saw a photographer. Disney made sure there were a ton of photographers, so I actually did run a good part of the race! There is nothing like 4 friends, some new, some who have not seen each other in years, getting together and enjoying the ability to catch up. Life is good.

If you know anything about the day before going on vacation, you know it is absolutely insane. The day before heading to Orlando, I had a doctor's appointment. Since I am Check2 positive, I needed to rule out any chances of melanoma. A cyst was found, and due to its location, I need to have it surgically removed. Also, they burned off some precancerous cells on my face while I was there. I found out that a check I sent to my credit card company was lost in the mail - I rarely use snail mail and right there justifies why. As I was on the phone with the credit card company paying off that bill (being that was the credit card the hotel had for our stay), the surgery center called trying to schedule the procedure. Well, since I did not answer immediately, they called my parents' house, being that they were my on my health records as "next of kin". Oh, the joys of being single....
"Mr. Boyd - we need to get Clara in for her surgical consult." Great - thanks for telling my dad before I could. And let's be honest - telling your dad you found a cyst on your ass on your 40th birthday not a priority in my life, but it became a priority when he then calls my mom,

freaking out and asking why I did not tell him I was having surgery. I can see it now – "Hey dad - you know what I want for Easter? A donut - as in something to sit on while my ass heals." Sigh This, plus preparing my company for my 4-day vacation, left me with what I thought was a migraine. I end up calling my dentist - ahhh the joys of living in a small town, your dentist gives you their cell phone number - I called her the night before vacation as the migraine that I thought I had moved down into my jaw. Really? Am I having a flipping heart attack or TMJ? I don't have time for either. I still have to pack all of my stuff for the trip, including my food, as I was partially on the Optifast food, and partially on real food. Fast forward to what she believed was TMJ. In all fairness, the symptoms I was relaying to her were that of TMJ. She told me what to do and said that if it got worse she would call in some Tylenol with codeine. I am a medical person, but not a pill person. I do not want to use prescriptions unless I have to. And the fact I was just taken off my metformin and blood pressure meds - I am not adding anything else in unless I need to.... this is foreshadowing at its finest....

Well, I make it until Wednesday morning before I am down for the count. I feel as if my face is on fire, and someone is using me as a punching bag. I signed up for a race - not 12 rounds with a professional boxer! I cannot lift my head off the pillow. Funny thing - it is just the right side of my face. The right side of my cheek, tongue, jaw, teeth, eye, etc. and it literally stopped in the middle of my face. With my medical background, I knew there was nerve involvement, but I am also stubborn - so in no way do I have time for this. My best friend, Val (another sister from another mister), who was on the trip called her dad Jay, who is an orthodontist. The same time I was having my dentist call in the codeine, Jay mentioned Trigeminal Neuralgia. Me, once again being stubborn, was not open to the fact that it would be this condition. His telltale words were – "If it is Trigeminal Neuralgia, the codeine won't touch it." What the hell does he mean by that? Codeine takes care of everything!?!? For me, codeine puts me on a whole other planet. I met my match. This thing packs a punch - pun intended. So, while I still had very viscous and vivid dreams - thanks codeine for my new nickname of Thrasher, it did not touch the pain.

Clara Boyd

There are many triggers for Trigeminal Neuralgia, but mine specifically are stress, eating and drinking. So, after the race I did not drink water, thus my system did not flush out the toxins. I go to weigh-in. For the first time in this whole process I gained weight. Three pounds to be exact. What the hell? Ironically, when I ran my half marathon I lost 3 pounds. I run a 5K and gain 3 pounds. Ugh. After the weigh in I end up at my primary care physician for the referral to the neurologist. Prior to the referral, she has decided to put me on prednisone for 2 weeks to calm everything down. Great prednisone - hello weight gain. Grrrr. Now we all know the rule of medicine. Don't go on the internet. Don't go on the internet. DON'T GO ON THE INTERNET!!!! I have a medical degree in health education. Do you know what that means? I know enough to know this is some serious shit. So, I start looking for peer-reviewed journals about Trigeminal Neuralgia. Guess how many I found...none. But I made my way to some internet sites that have me freaked out. Plan of attack prednisone for 2 weeks to calm everything down. Next up CT scan, or MRI. Then, anti-seizure meds for life. FOR LIFE! I just got off all of my meds. Ugh. A dear friend asked me if this is because I lost the weight so quickly. One of the theories is actually the precancerous cells that were frozen of my face were so close to one of the branches of the nerve, that the nerve was nicked. Great. But in the end who knows? It doesn't really matter, I have to put my big girl pants on and deal with this. So ultimately, the cyst on my rear is nothing compared to the cells on my face. Worst case scenario is brain surgery. You can bet your sweet tushie I will be researching the hell out of the doctors that perform the surgery and how necessary it really is.

With all of this being said, I am leaving today for Cape Cod for 2 weeks. Val lives there, and her dad is the orthodontist. Jay is my second dad, "Dad 2" as I lovingly call him. I feel good that if I have an emergency while I am there I will be OK. I have my prednisone in hand, and I am leaving on a jet plane! So, the fear returns this is the first trip since I lost the weight. Will I fit into the seat? Will I need a seatbelt extender? Come on - this entry started with a fairytale theme, it ends with it too.

Sitting in the seat comfortably - no extender needed. God is good. I am good. This crazy journey we call life is amazing.

All of my love ~ Clara

March 7, 2017 – Facebook

ATC/PT/medical friends... What do we know about Trigeminal Neuralgia? Any peer-reviewed info out there? Best neurosurgeon for procedure? Asking for a friend. Starting my research today. Thanks in advance.

Asking for a friend – I was not going to let the cat out of the bag just yet that I may or may not be having brain surgery. This was on my mind, literally and figuratively. This was all I could think about. Scary enough, a friend from high school reached out to me as she had previously dealt with the same situation and ultimately had to have the surgery. If nothing else, I knew I could reach out to her for advice.

March 12, 2017 – Private Thoughts

Simon and Garfunkel could always express life in an amazing way in my opinion. "Homeward Bound" by them was the song always came on, on my way home from Clemson every trip. I am not in a railway station, but the Charlotte airport. Have you ever noticed how many rocking chairs this place has? My former boss mentioned it one time, and that is all I can see now. The rocking chair industry loves this place for sure! I am homeward bound after 13 days on the Cape. There is nothing like being with a friend that knows more about you than you do yourself! As a reminder to her, I know her pretty darn well too. My job allows me to be flexible, and I was able to work while I was there. So, she would go to work daily, and I would work at her home - then we would enjoy the evenings reminiscing and making new memories.

I love how people that are in your life for the right reasons support you. Like really support you. Val is one of those people - never there to coerce but will tell you when you are going off your path. I was able to stay on track with my diet this trip. We would go for coffee on a daily basis -

Clara Boyd

Cape Cod has Dunks like Carter has liver pills (Which by the way - my mom used to always say that - did President Carter have a liver problem?) Anywho - there was never pressure to cheat, but coffee to me was my treat, so I felt as if I was getting a treat on a daily basis. I would eat my bar for breakfast, yogurt for snack, salad with deli turkey on top for lunch, fruit for snack, and then dinner (3 oz protein and a veggie!)

Here is my problem with losing weight when you are on vacation - especially a 13-day vacation. The airlines allow one bag at $25.00 And then the price goes up. I am Dutch - Let me tell you how much I can pack into one suitcase - and yes - it was right at 50 pounds. We are digressing. I lost weight on vacation, which meant my clothes were not fitting by the end. I am sitting here in a pair of jeans that fit nicely 14 days ago, and they are falling off me now. This is an amazing problem to have! The seat belt on the first flight had about 6 inches of extra seat belt around it. This is an amazing problem too - that I have not seen since college days! So, my size 20 jeans get washed tonight, and donated. The size 18 will be donated in a few weeks. The majority of the clothes I packed for this trip did not fit by the end of the trip. Size 16 (and 14) jeans are already ordered.

My face problems got worse this week. I will be seeing a doctor in Gainesville on Wednesday. They started the anti-seizure meds a week ago. Is it weird that all I can smell is pot? Is that a side effect? Hmmmm. The next step is surgery where they perform a craniotomy, stick a sponge in my head between the nerve and the blood vessel that is annoying it. Ummmm - really? That is the best fix? However I am not going to fight with this man. I ended up finding a few peer-reviewed journal articles about Trigeminal Neuralgia, and damn it - this really sucks! This surgery has an 85% success rate. If someone told me I had an 85% chance of winning the lottery, I would double up! So why not? He is also the best in the Southeast. So - to Gator land I go.

Val and I do have a way of finding ourselves off the beaten path. Literally and figuratively. When we both lived in Tallahassee - years ago - before smart phones, we went for a walk. And on this walk, we found a bike path. This bike path led to a road, and next thing you know we were an hour into this walk, with no clue where we were. We finally had come to a neighborhood. I called my sister in a panic, as we are tired and a little scared. She said they would come to pick us up immediately. She asked where we were. I told her I don't know! To spare you all the details, we finally figured we were about 4 miles away from my house. My sister, her husband, and the kids were on their way to a friend's house for a birthday party. My nieces were really young at this point, so they had the car seats from hell. Kim and Rob were in the front seat, so that left Val and I sitting in the bed of the truck on top of the coolers. It was either that or the Princess car that the kids drove.

Getting back to this past week. Every year, I have a physical goal that I challenge myself with. Last year was to run a half marathon. This year was to try yoga. Val was so excited because she found a Yoga studio. She signed us up and we were going until we were supposed to go. We ended up looking for a couch that night instead. Val knew that taking my mind off of the fear of potential brain surgery by laughing and looking for a couch is a lot more important than making it to the yoga class.

Let me tell you about this couch. Double recliner, power head rest, dark brown leather. Let's just say that the majority of my time in the house after that purchase included loung- ing on that couch. Getting off the beaten path can be fun and relaxing, especially when it involves that couch.

I said goodbye to Val today, knowing I will see her in June, and I promised the couch I would be back too.

Back to reality, and back to a weigh in in the morning.

All of my love ~ Clara

March 15, 2017 - Facebook

Clara Boyd

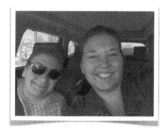

This picture was taken after I met with the neurosurgeon, Dr. Friedman at University of Florida. At this point, the anti-seizure meds would not allow me to form full sentences as I could not clearly speak. I had words in my head, but I could not get them to my mouth.

This still happens to this day, but not nearly as much. I remember the frustration, and thinking – what kind of quality of life is this? When meeting with the neurosurgeon, he im- mediately realized the severity, and scheduled the surgery for 6 days later. Thankfully we were able to do pre-op that day since I lived two hours away. The memory from that day that always sticks out in my mind is the memory of meeting with anesthesiology. The doctor asked me if I used a CPAP machine. I could not lie to him. This was brain surgery!

There are times that we may tell doctors little white lies. Do I lie to my dentist about how often I floss? Of course! Then the morning before my dental appointment I floss really well and brush my teeth really REALLY well! This was not the time to lie. I fessed up and told them that I was not using my CPAP any more as the machine felt like I was standing in front of a wind tunnel. I had lost so much weight that I did not need it anymore. The anesthesiologist was so proud of me and praised me for my hard work. He told me that it was quite impressive. While I was so proud of my accomplishment, it still did not calm my fears for the upcoming surgery. Just make sure I wake up from this, please God....

March 17, 2017 – Facebook

When life gives you lemons - go cut your hair!

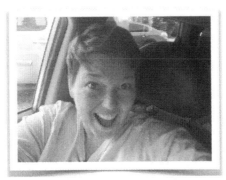

<u>*Wow if I do not look like my picture from Chapter 1! (Go back and look, it's ok, I just did too!)*</u>

Man – talk about people private messaging you wondering why you cut your hair – Did you break up with a boyfriend? What is going on? Boyd gals look cute with short hair (which **we do, by the way...**)

Time to privately tell people what is going on. I want to be in control of who knows what. I do NOT want a pity party, I need to be in control. Goodness – I am not in control of many things right now, maybe I can be in control of who knows about this brain surgery…

<u>March 17, 2017 – Facebook</u>

There's that word again…. Badass it would make for a great tattoo I hear. Lol

When I let a dear friend know what was happening, she called me a Badass. I don't have any tattoos. There is a lot of commitment with a tattoo and I am too scared. But I was about to have brain surgery. I will take the nickname of Badass. Thank you.

<u>March 19, 2017 – Private Thoughts</u>

Tomorrow morning, I have my final weigh-in for the program. So many thoughts going thru my head, very little of them about the weigh-in. I have maintained my program for 18 weeks. I have done what I am supposed to, including losing 10.5 pounds on vacation. Woo hoo!!! Not only are the size 20s getting donated. So are the size 18s! I

Clara Boyd

am in a size 16 again. Down 8 sizes. I have not been in a size 16 since Beyoncé was one of Destiny's children and 50 cent had a stick that was magical. This week though for the final weigh-in... I have no clue where I will be. I have been on anti-seizure meds for over 2 weeks now due to the Trigeminal Neuralgia. I have kept to my diet, but how will these meds affect me? I am drinking water like a fish. I have concluded after this Wednesday - it is what it is. This past Wednesday I traveled to Gainesville to Shands to see Dr. Friedman, a neurosurgeon that specializes in Trigeminal Neuralgia. After an evaluation from his resident and him, it was decided that I need to go ahead and have the surgery. This particular surgery places a sponge in my head to separate the blood vessel and the nerve. They ruled out multiple sclerosis and a tumor thank goodness! All I can think of this whole time is Arnold in one of his best performances "Kindergarten Cop" – and that I don't have a tumah! To rule it out was an MRI. Have you ever had an MRI on your head? They put a "Silence of the Lamb" style mask over your face, and then place you in the tube for 45 minutes. I have had one in the past; that is when I figured out I was claustrophobic. Thus, when they started this MRI, I decided to close my eyes. Going into the tube, I could feel my shoulders hitting the sides of the tube. They lifted up the table, and then I could feel my arms on the top of the tube. The whole 45 minutes all I could think was - thank goodness I have lost 67 pounds. How in the hell would I have fit in the tube? Well, after the MRI, blood work, pharmacy, and meeting the anesthesiologist, we were on our way back home.

The last couple days have been a blur. My mom is my rock. I love both of my parents, and all of my family, but my mom is the matriarch, and everyone knows it. She has taken over for me. Even to the point of driving me. Yesterday I gave up driving. The meds that I am on are increasingly impairing my thoughts and abilities. There are words in my brain that I cannot get to my mouth, I have short term memory loss, and now driving is just not even worth attempting. Not that she would have it any other way, but she has taken control - organizing my paperwork for the hospital, including insurance, FMLA, and all other paperwork; my prescriptions, including the hibaclens soap, *and the stuff I am swabbing my nose with. On Friday, we talked about cutting my hair. Let me preface this with I am not one of these girls that believes you need to have long hair to be feminine. Many beautiful women I know have short hair. This is coming down to the fact that I am not in control of anything. I am getting a little pissed off - I have no option on this surgery. It is called the suicide disease as many people killed themselves prior to the development of this surgery due to the pain. I need someone else to be in control of me because I cannot take care of myself. My hair is the one thing I could have control over. Until we talked about it on Friday morning. One of the number one postoperative problem is infection in the incision. Being that they are shaving part of my head, I wanted to be in control of how I would have to deal with my hair. Short pixie was the way to go.*

2 days in ICU throwing up (nausea is one of the problems post-op) and then home in bed for 2 weeks. I can work out in 6 weeks. Lord knows that was my first question to the doctor.

I know I will do great on Tuesday. I don't have a choice in it. And I already have my outfit picked out for Halloween - Bride of Frankenstein. And I may have a new style ;)

All of my love ~ Clara

March 20, 2017 – Facebook

In 18 weeks, I have lost 70 pounds. I am officially finished with the program, and in maintenance. To say I have a new lease on life is an understatement. I did it the healthy way. I cannot thank the TMH Bariatric Center enough! Check them out if you are serious about losing weight.

I wrote that post on my way out of town heading south to Gainesville for brain surgery early the next morning. Funny thing, you would think I would celebrate with a cheeseburger, or pasta, or a typical comfort food that I used to run to, especially as nervous as I was on the inside. Nope. I had a turkey sandwich that night as Mom and I had bigger plans. Hometown hero,

David Ross was going to be on *Dancing with the Stars*, and we needed to find our hotel in time to make sure we watched him dance. Priorities, people. Priorities. Furthermore, I still have a long way to go on this weight loss journey – Tuesday was going to be "Just a little brain surgery". That's all...

March 23, 2017 – Facebook

Alright - I was not going to say anything on Facebook, but here I sit reading the negativity, and I am truly disgusted as to what people are complaining about. (Also a few friends leaked out the information by mistake)

Tuesday, I had brain surgery at Shands. This is not a joke. Apparently, surgery went great, recovery did not go as smooth. Things I have learned in the last 50 hours of my life...

#1 - They did find a brain in there

#2 - I am an overachiever - instead of 1 blood vessel wrapped around the nerve, I had 2 blood vessels wrapped around this nerve

#3 - I have the best friends and family anyone could ever wish for. I can never thank all of you enough.

#4 - Shands is amazing, and I am officially a Gator fan. Thank you to their neurosurgeons and their staff.

#5 All of this petty BS that people complain on FB about-it's exactly that - BS.

Enjoy life, you never know when you are faced with something as serious as this. I am not asking for the obligatory 'Hope you feel better'. I am not seeking attention. I would much rather you post something happy instead of negative the next time you are on FB. And with that one of my dearest friends would say I have sunshine flowing from me. He is right.

But this is why I cut my hair (and I heard from my nieces that I am stylish to have half of my head shaved! Lights are still bothering me so I will not be checking FB or out and about for the next 3 weeks or so. I am going to comply with the doctor and rest like I am supposed to. I will however accept all prayers that you have to offer.

All of my love - Clara

March 29, 2017 – Facebook

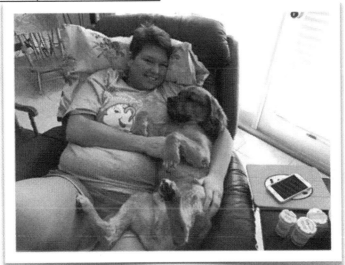

My nurse, Tramp. He is taking a break, apparently.

Tramp, our dog. He has many names, but the best is "Tramp the Wonder Dog". Tramp, you may have guessed, was named after the movie *Lady and the Tramp*. While he looks more like Lady he is a male, so he was named Tramp. We rescued him from the pound, but like all rescues you always wonder, who really rescued who? He is a really good nurse as most dogs are. I was eight days post-op at this point and very frustrated with many things, one of them being that I could not exercise. Who would have thought I would have such an addiction? I was worried about my weight loss, my food intake, and my lack of exercise.

The shirt I am wearing in this picture is from the 5K I did at Walt Disney World in February before surgery. I needed any sort of inspiration to stay positive. Light and sound was still bothering me. I was sleeping the majority of the time, and when I was awake I had a constant migraine. However, I wanted to exercise – that is all I wanted to do and I could not. I was frustrated, damn it.

Clara Boyd

April 3, 2017 – Facebook

My sister sent me a saying this morning about a mountain I have been assigned to show others that it can be moved. Could relate to a few things in my life right now. Just left the doctor. Lost 5.5 pounds this week amidst healing. I miss my workouts. I miss my daily walks. I miss my work - especially my friends that are also my coworkers. Life is not normal right now but getting closer every day. Love to all of you.

April 23, 2017 – Private Thoughts

For the past month I have felt like the scarecrow. I needed a brain. Well, I needed to fix my brain. So - I ended up going to Shands. I had hit the 70 pound mark the day before surgery, so I was truly happy with my weight at that point. I weighed in at 250 pounds. I went to my weekly group meeting, and then on the road to Gainesville for surgery.

Surgery and the next few days were a blur. I ended up having 2 blood vessels touching the nerve, thus, it ended up being a much more intense surgery than anticipated. I must commend the neurosurgery medical staff at Shands. I feel blessed that the research was done and they knew exactly how to fix my broken head. There are a few things that I remember about the day of surgery. Pre-op is very efficient. They called about 10 of us back at one time, and then divided us up into pre-op beds. I had a very nice pre-op nurse. Waiting for the anesthesiologist to come into my curtained partition area, I watched all the hot anes- thesiologists start to assist the other patients. When my anesthesiologist finally arrived, he was at least 60, with a Latin accent. He was a sweet little old man - almost wanted to ask him to drink a cafe con leche with me and chat - not oversee my breathing for the next 4 hours. But I was rewarded. The resident surgeon was different from the one I saw for pre-op. This guy was handsome - like Clark Kent who worked out - WOWZERS. I was so nervous, he explained everything to me, and then it was time to go. I was wheeled into the OR. I was so nervous that tears were coming out of my eyes, landing on the pillow beneath me. When I got into the OR, I tried to be funny and wink at my Superman (or in my brain at least he was mine...lol) But I did not find comfort in his smile.

Losing One Hundred Pounds

Do you know who comforted me? You guessed it. My cafe con leche buddy. While they were preparing me for surgery - people at every appendage, strapping me down, adding leg massagers onto my lower legs, getting ready to put my head in a vice (YES - my head was literally put in a vice! Bad thing about that - my dad offered to do the surgery out in the garage with a shot of whiskey and putting my head in the vice on his workbench and I told him he was crazy - maybe he is not!); out of nowhere I feel someone grab my left hand. I still had tears streaming down my face, as I tried to act brave. I look over, and the sweet cafe con leche anesthesiologist says to me - "I've got you - I will take care of you, I promise." And with that - I knew I was in good hands. I truly believe that God puts people in places when you need them. I believe to LET GO AND LET GOD. I did let go and peacefully allowed God to be in control. Within 24 hours of surgery, I was up and walking. In fact - walking the halls. At one point - a nurse remarked "There she goes again" in a positive tone. I looked at her and remarked - I am getting the hell up out of here! Not the nicest of responses, but I will use the excuse that I just had brain surgery. :)

The next 3 weeks were filled with a lot of sleep and constant migraines. I am still having daily migraines, but the severity and length are decreasing. I do need to laugh though. I craved scallops and tangerines. I had both daily - and I did not care. I wanted scallops anyway I could get them. It makes me think of the movie "Forrest Gump" - when Bubba talked about all the different ways you could cook shrimp but insert scallops. You would think that this would be great for my weight. It was not bad, but it wasn't good. I have maintained my weight for the last month. One week I am 249.5 and the next 250.0 Many people thought that when I ended the transition program, I would gain the weight back. For a month I have been steady at 250. So, of that - I am proud.

I went back to work this week. Slow and steady wins the race - that is what people have told me about going back to work. I agree with them. I am glad to return to work. I like normalcy, and work is a major part of that. With all of this being said - tomorrow starts a new week. Back to my lifestyle changes and to a healthier me.

Clara Boyd

All of my love

~ Clara

June 11, 2017 – Facebook

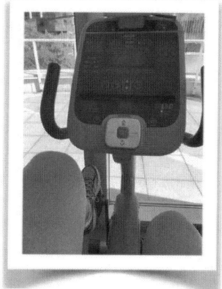

Because even on vacation, I have to answer to my trainer, and more importantly. Myself! Weights up next! (I may have to fight off a polar bear!)

Improving yourself never takes a vacation – even when you are on vacation! We were about to go on an Alaskan cruise. It is true what they say – going on a cruise, there are food temptations everywhere! Thank goodness I worked out daily. There was a gym on the ship, and the trainers knew my name by day two, so I think that is a good sign. I still gained 12 pounds on an 8-day cruise – YIKES! There is a balance for sure – I did not do too well.

However, I did enjoy myself.

June 16, 2017 – Facebook

Because life is about living on the lines. Alaska zip.

There are things in life that scare you – brain surgery, zip-lining, losing weight, and finding yourself. I had never zip-

Losing One Hundred Pounds

lined before. It may sound silly but I feel very secure if my feet are on a platform. Without a platform, I lose my sense of being in control. A great example of this is Soarin' at Walt Disney's EPCOT – It is a hang-gliding experience-type movie ride. There is a screen in front of you, a huge fan blowing wind in your face to give you the feeling that you are hang gliding. Are you really hang gliding? No, but it is Disney – so it magically transports you into that wonderful world. But I am cold and clammy for the mere fact that my feet are not on a platform. I am not in control.

When you zip-line, your feet, are obviously not on a platform. At the point that we are zip-lining in Alaska, I had bravely lost approximately 75 pounds, had brain surgery, battled many emotional aspects of both of these feats, and I am terrified to let go of this platform. As I am watching my family, one by one let go of the platform, my fear intensifies. My brother-in-law, a firefighter, who does this all the time goes first; he of course has no fear. My oldest niece, Taylor – no fear. My dad – retired firefighter – no fear. My youngest niece, Alex - it is her turn. At this point, the zip-lining guide reiterates to all of us in the group that there are two cables – one will hold 750+ pounds of pressure and one will hold 1500+ pounds of pressure. Now, I ate a few desserts during the cruise, but I knew the cables would hold. My niece Alex goes – no fear; my sister Kim goes – no fear. My mom, needs a little nudge to go, as she has a bit of a hesitation – but at 66, and 8 weeks after her second knee replacement – she is zip-lining.

And now it is my time to go – Clip. Clip. My harnesses are attached to both of the cables. It is my turn to let go. My every instinct is yelling at me to walk back off this ledge! Walk back down the stairs, back down to the lodge, drink a few beers and wait for the rest of the family. Sure, they might be angry at first, but there is a lot of zip-lining to do before they would see me again. That's a ton of time for them to cool down, right? I know if I start zip-lining – I am not in control. Even though it is misty and cool, I am dripping sweat as my nerves are getting the best of me. I am not in control. I cannot control this situation. I can't control the zip-line.

I can hear the guide telling me to bend my knees, sit down and JUST lift my knees. My mouth and throat are so dry I cannot even speak to say anything to her. I am thinking - "Shut up, woman. I am not in control then." She is positively coercing me and encouraging me, and I am still thinking I can still go back to the lodge. Years of worry and doubt are rushing through my mind - starting a goal and never finishing it because of fear, whether it was losing weight or a fitness goal. This cyclical negative experience was coming right back like it always did. I could walk away from this experience, from life, or I could find peace and let go.

While I still have these negative thoughts, a calming peace came over me. Why won't I just LET GO? CLARA – JUST LET GO! That was all I needed. I bent my knees, sat down, lifted my knees... and LET GO. Freedom! My eyes were glued shut for the majority of the first zip-line, hands clenched tight to the bar, and I am pretty sure I did not breathe either. Once I opened my eyes, only one word could describe my flight thought the Alaskan wilderness – Majestic. The scenery was stunning. Green and vibrant, a canopy of trees with rivers running through them – absolutely breathtaking. Before I knew it – the first zip-line was done. The lead guide needed to catch me after the first zip-line as I was too scared to let go of the bar, but with each zip-line my confidence grew. What was I so scared of originally? I could not even remember anymore. I even started smiling, enjoying myself, and assisted the lead by grabbing other zip-liners when they would get to the next platform. By the final zip-line, I leaped off the platform backwards, my eyes wide open, arms and legs extended out, falling backwards into the wilderness letting go of all inhibitions and fears, and I was finally able to exhale. It was more than just zip-lining at that point, I was letting go of so many fears. I was going to start living. Life was good, and I was living it, out loud. I found peace in LETTING GO!

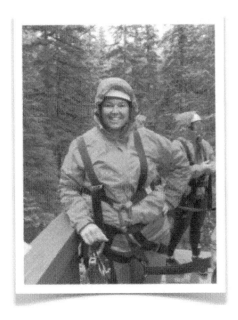

July 13, 2017 – Private Thoughts

For as many years that I have been alive, my birthday has been a great day. First off - it is in the middle of the summer. As a kid - I loved it - I NEVER had to go to school on my birthday, I had a pool party (although I was jealous of my sister who used to have Chuck E Cheese parties as her birthday is in November), AND I share my birthday with one helluva hottie - Harrison Ford, or as I like to remember him fondly - Indiana Jones (I still wonder how he got the scar on his chin???). I fondly remember calling my friend's mom
on my birthday, and when she answered I said, "Mrs. Stevens - it is your idol's birthday!" With that I got a slap on the top of my head from my grandma - back when you were disciplined for mouthing off - Mrs. Stevens was in love with Harrison Ford, and of course I meant him and not me. Once I explained it, Grandma and I had a great laugh together.
Mrs. Stevens also reminds me to this day that I fell out of her Dodge Ram Charger head first when she was dropping me off at elementary school one day. She could not even ask if I was OK, as she was laughing

so hard she was crying. 30+ years later, we still laugh about that experience today.

Even with all those fond memories, since I was a teenager and old enough to be concerned with what others thought, I have not woken up truly HAPPY on my birthday. There was always some regret; something I knew I had to work on. Mainly my weight. I wish I had lost weight, I wish I was a size 8 like my friends, I wish that boy liked me - I just KNOW he would if I was skinnier, etc. As I woke up last year in Aruba on my 40th birthday, I was sad. As I opened my eyes I thought, "Here I am - 40 years old and 326 pounds." (Probably even more as we really enjoyed ourselves at the bars that week.) I was not HAPPY. I should have been HAPPY. There are many people that do not ever see Aruba, and what is more important, many that do not see 40 years old! I am so selfish for having these thoughts when I have so much to be thankful for.

But that was last year... The journey I have been on this year has taught me a lot. From the daily struggle and triumph over my weight, to the brain surgery, I have taken a look both inward and outward. I have looked inside me to see who I am and who I want to be professionally and personally.

Professionally, I decided to shift my goals. I have always wanted to climb all the way up the corporate ladder, and there is nothing wrong with that, however, there really is nothing wrong with NOT climbing all the way to the top. (Please note - in my opinion - there is nothing wrong with climbing that ladder. I 100% support my friends, family, and peers that are taking it step by step.) With everything that happened this year, starting with the thyroid biopsy, my life focuses have shifted. I have stopped climbing that ladder and have stayed pretty much lateral professionally. You know what? It is not too bad! Is there stress? Sure! Am I HAPPY? Absolutely! I have found my HAPPY place professionally. I love my team, I love our struggles, as we focus on them together to find solutions, and I love our successes. My professional life is right where I want it to be for now. At the end of the day, are we who we are because of our profession, or is there more to us?

I thought about how I treated others. Am I the best friend I can be? Am I the best daughter, sister, aunt? Am I giving others all of me, or just enough to keep them where I need them? Am I HAPPY with myself? If you have read any part of this journey, you know that I am getting HAPPIER every day, as I am working on myself every day. Physically, I am getting HAPPIER - hell, I even took a gym selfie today - which I never do. Who does that? I guess people that are either justifying to others that they work out, or HAPPY gym people.

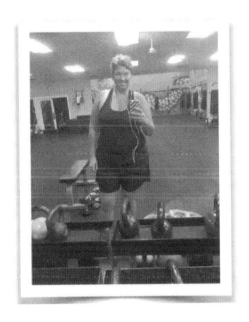

I remember about 8 years ago wanting to work out on my birthday. I remember texting my trainer asking if I should workout. It was my birthday and all, so - what a better way to start the day than with a workout. He never responded, so I never went. What the hell? Why was it his job to get me to go to the gym? I was not HAPPY with going to the gym, but I wanted to make it sound like I was. He did the best thing he could do - he called me out on it. He told me if I wanted to be there, I would have been. I started my day today at the gym, and no one needed to tell me to do it, I was HAPPY to. I want to make sure that I am the best friend, daughter, sister, aunt I can be - and that starts with making my-

self HAPPY.

*Making myself HAPPY - oh - there are things I still need to do to make that truly happen. but how do we measure that? What does that truly mean? There is this perception that I keep coming back to - if I was married/dating a guy. If I was out of financial debt and independently wealthy. And then I picked up a book. "The Subtle Art of Not Giv-ing a F*ck." I know - WOW! What a name! I highly recommend it. Read it - even if you are not a reader. (By the way - I find it ironic that I am writing this journal as someone who HATED reading as a kid - Cliff was my best friend - as in Cliff Notes.) Although I want you to read this book, and my journal of course, I will give you the very basic summary - Focus on what you really care about in life, give a F*ck about those things and let everything else take care of itself. Even easier than that - Not your circus, not your monkeys! Would I like to be married? Yes - but then would he be HAPPY if I spent the summer on Cape Cod? Would I like to be independently wealthy? Yes - but would I be HAPPY if...wait - yes, I would be HAPPY. It would allow for me to really focus on what I want in life - maybe volunteer somewhere, maybe hop in the RV and just go - who knows?*

What makes us HAPPY is different for each and every one. Last night I sat at a high-top table at a bar and listened to an 88-year-old woman talk about the Cape Cod Baseball League. See, these "boys" are the best of the best college baseball players, and they are housed by local families during their summer time here on the Cape. "Mrs. E" has housed players longer than I have been alive, and being a spry 88-year-old, she can remember each and every one of them. Stories about them, their families, and their major league careers. As the hours passed, and I was trying to keep my eyes open (I cannot remember the last time I was out that late) she continued to tell their stories. The glimmer in her eyes - she was in her HAPPY place. All I could think was - I hope that in 47 years, I am sitting on a bar stool reminiscing about the good ol' days and I am as HAPPY today as I was back then. She has enjoyed this journey, and I know when she goes to the big bullpen in the sky (her words, not mine) she will be HAPPY that she lived her life.

I love that I am finding my HAPPINESS - everyday. I have forgiven those that have tried to take away my HAPPINESS. I have forgiven myself for those times I have tried to take away my own HAPPINESS. I look forward to the journey in finding and optimizing my HAPPINESS. This journey included zip-lining on a family cruise to Alaska and learning to let go of my need to control. Remember my mention of Soarin'? I get clammy hands and do all I can not to cry as my nieces are holding my hands as they know how nervous I get. With my feet firmly planted on the ground, I am in control. But in control of what? Certainly not my HAPPINESS. There is something to be said about letting go - stepping off that platform and just LETTING GO! I found my HAPPINESS strapped to a harness flying over treetops in a rainforest in Juneau, Alaska.

The zip-line trail was filled with inspirational quotes including Dale Carnegie's infamous quote, and I paraphrase - about putting off living, dreaming of a rose garden elsewhere and not enjoying the roses that are right around us. Whatever your HAPPINESS, find it, embrace it, and live it! This morning, for the first time in 30+ years, on July 13th - I woke up HAPPY...with no regrets.

July 16, 2017 – Facebook

Just finished my 1st hot yoga session. Very intense. A little addictive. Need to find a place in Tallahassee. Any thoughts?

Val does not forget about my goals... Remember from March? She let me have a pass in March because of the brain surgery back then, but she was not going to now. Yeah... We were going to fulfill this goal. Sigh. Yoga. Hot yoga. Have you ever taken the class? If you have not, try it. It is amazing. Let me set the scene. It feels like you are walking into the Sahara on in the middle of July, and they are having a heat wave, with 99.9% humidity. Remember how I mentioned Val and I have this way of find ourselves in the middle of an adventure? We did, yet again. For our first class, we started with a 90-minute session. First class ever. 90 minutes. Sahara dessert. I believe the room was set to around 100 degrees. On the cool side of this topic, everyone was so supportive and nice. I think they took pity on me really, as they saw the fear on my face.

Val is an athletic goddess who kept up with the class, as she has done yoga in the past. I have too, in the comfort of my home, on my tablet. You know – a couple quick stretches – I was such the "yoga expert". A little Namaste here, a little Savasana there. But a legit yoga class – I had never done one. I was more like a yoga novice.

Great. Here we go. At least I had a spot by the window so that I could look out of it and dream what I could be doing other than bending like a pretzel. Within the first minute I was sweating. Within two minutes, I had so much sweat in my eyes, I could not see out of that window I was right next to. I kept praying please don't fall please don't fall. I don't want to look like an idiot – just don't fall flat on your face, Boyd. Just don't fall flat on your face! There was a sweet man next to me that talked me through the entire class. Thank goodness for him. He was doing his good deed for the day. Hot yoga is so hot, that I literally was wringing my clothes out during the class. I was wondering if I had any water left in me at all! The humidity in the class was so intense by the end, that the instructor came by with about 3 minutes left to crack the window. My window – I picked the perfect spot! I knew I would never see these people again, and there was no shame in my game. We were kneeling at this point, and I climbed up the wall, looking like Mel Brooks as President Skroob in *Spaceballs* inhaling the oxygen out of the can when she opened the window. Fresh cool air! I am so glad I completed that class. Yoga really is an amazing workout. I like it…maybe next time, I will just leave the hot out of the yoga.

August 14, 2017 – Facebook

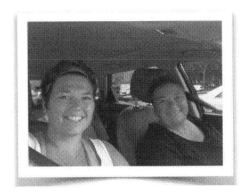

Post-Gym Selfie

Since everyone else is posting their first day of school pics, here is ours! I got "schooled" by my mom when I got to the gym and she had already been on the treadmill for 15 minutes without me. Way to go mom!

Hope everyone had an amazing first day! I enjoyed seeing all of your babies growing up!

You are never too old to get schooled by your mom. I am so proud of her. We have been working out together for 6 years now at this point. While there are days that we still need that motivation/accountability from the other to get to the gym, those days are few and far between. There are many more days that we are so excited to workout that we are encouraging each other by trying new machines, new workout routines, or pushing each other in a positive way. Having the perfect workout partner can make all the difference in the world!

August 20, 2017 – Personal Thoughts

There is a meme going around social media showing a scale in a doctor's office and it discusses being offended by it. Why are we so stuck on what the scale says? And I am including myself in that "WE". Why are we so stuck on numbers? Is it a competition? Do we have to be the best? Do we have to always "one up" someone? Are we not enough unless we have reached a certain goal? What is really important – what is more important – the number on the scale or the numbers in my bloodwork?

There is a fine line. 326 is not healthy, I know this. But there is a certain point where the numbers in my bloodwork are going to be a lot more important than the scale. I need to find this balance and be happy.

September 4, 2017 – Facebook

Hurricane Irma is on her way, UGH! OK. I am sticking to my diet somehow. But - there are a lot of temptations in this house.

Floridians know that Mother Nature is going to send storms out way. Tallahassee was hit by Irma, but she was so weak by the time she hit us, we were spared the worst. Sadly, that is not always the case with hurricanes, and there was still damage and secondary concerns such as power outages. These stressors cause changes into routines and diet and exercise. Sometimes we can control the stressors, and sometimes it is a hurricane challenge! When the power goes out you go into survival mode, and everyone knows ice cream thaws a lot faster than broccoli! In all seriousness, I am reminded of Maslow's Hierarchy of Needs. We are concerned with our basic physiological needs – food, shelter, and water; and not self-actualization – reaching full potential. Focusing on basic needs are more important than en- suring that we are focused on our goals. It is OK. Give yourself a break.

September 7, 2017 – Facebook

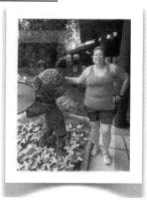

Two years ago, today. Wow - how time flies and weight drops. This is 80 pounds ago.

Timehop…while I am typically not a big fan, when losing weight it can be a great reminder of where you have been and is a great reminder of why you are doing what you are doing!

October 19, 2017 – Facebook

Shout out to Academy Sports. They have recognized that women of all sizes workout. While I am slimming myself right out of this section, it is nice to see that there is finally a section for women of ALL sizes to purchase legitimate workout gear. Let me know if you need some design/style ideas. #BigGirlsWorkoutToo

Do you know how hard it is to find workout clothes in plus size for women? Within the past year, it is getting easier. However, I have always found it ironic, that it is easy to find men's workout clothes in plus sizes up to 6X, etc., but finding a 3X or 4X in a women's is far and few between. Even online! Major companies are starting to recognize this. When I went to my first race expo, I was hoping to purchase some race T-shirts. I was excited and went to the official company that was sponsoring the event. The largest size they offered for ladies was XL. When I asked a representative where the ladies plus sizes were located, they looked dumb founded. I looked her straight in the eyes and said – Big Girls Run Too! I told her that this is a market they are sorely missing out on, and that they were missing out on a major profit. Now, I am not saying that I am the reason that they changed their mind, but two years later, at the same expo, they have plus sizes through 3X. We have progress being made.

While we are on the subject of clothes, I have never had much fashion sense. How could I? While there have been "Plus Size" or "Women" areas in department stores for years, fashion-able, affordable, plus size clothing is a different story. I enjoyed shopping at Lane Bryant, but on a teacher's salary, I bought clothes there typically on clearance or solid tops and pants so that I could mix and match my outfits. Being in athletics I usually had to wear athletic shorts and T-shirts anyway, so I ended up being in sweats most of the time. Working for a high school, the athletic department ordered the clothes in bulk, which meant all the clothes that were ordered were mens apparel. I was looking so fashionable.

All that changed when I scored my job working remotely from my house. For a girl with no fashion sense, I feel like I just won the lottery wearing T-shirt and shorts EVERYDAY! Until the day arrives when you go to visit the Governor's mansion and meet the First Lady, Ann Scott. Wait, what? First Lady Scott is a literacy advocate and a person of great importance in the Florida educational scene. For my company, it was requested that I join the meet and greet. At the point of this happening, I was back to a size 14 already, but do not own any clothes appropriate to meet the First Lady of the State. Since I planned to lose more weight, I could not justify spending a lot of money on dressy clothes as I work from home. So, shopping I would go. I walked into The Loft. Great store, very nice employees. While I was browsing the racks, I began a conversation with one of them, and she politely asks me about my style. My style??? What the heck is she talking about? What is MY STYLE? My style has always been whatever I can fit in, and it won't split or tear if I sit down. Something I will still be able to breathe in; nothing with buttons, as they will pop off; and please…. nothing with 100% cotton as that will shrink – so if that is a style, that is it!

While I was screaming that inside, I was too embarrassed to say it, so I quietly said – I don't know. She looked at me like I had two heads, and then I confessed – I just lost a lot of weight, and the last time I shopped for a dress I was a size 26. Her eyes welled with tears, she immediately grabbed two other women, and I became their project. I felt like Julia Roberts in *Pretty Woman* when she was on Rodeo Drive the second time around, minus the whole "Pretty Woman profession". I was being draped with dresses and showered with compliments. It was the first time in my life I enjoyed shopping. Ever.

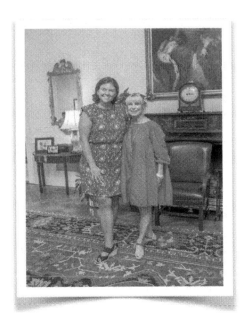

Me and First Lady Ann Scott. Such a privilege to meet her. (Photographer, Brittany Clark)

October 21, 2017 – Facebook

What do you do in Tallahassee when your team has a bye week? Go to the gym of course! Nobody's there :) Now off to watch some really good football for the day with no stress of winning or losing. Go Tigers!

No excuses – even during the most wonderful time of the year.

October 31, 2017 – Facebook

Alright - to say I am addicted to races is an understatement. But this one is going to be insane. Yes - I am challenging myself - but for a great cause! Who wants to run it with me and a dear friend of mine? (OK - let's be honest, we walk unless we see a photographer or the finish line.) Join us for a great cause, three days of challenging yourself, and a fun time in one of the greatest states in the union!

My sisters from other misters – they challenge me in such positive ways. Laura and I signed up for a 3-day 30-mile race to raise money for Breast Cancer. Holy crap! This one was going to challenge me emotionally, mentally, and physically. What did I get myself into? There is a much bigger battle out there. Much bigger than me – I needed to quit being selfish – and I put one step in front of the other.

November 3-4, 2017

My race addiction has now spilled over into my family. My mom, the matriarch of the family has always taken care of everyone else. Since retirement in 2016, my mom had a few health setbacks, which may have stopped many people from achieving their goals; but being the strong woman that she is, she was not going to let these health issues bring her down.
Two new knees later, mom was ready to tackle her first 5K race. She too has been on this weight loss journey with me. It was because she needed a knee replacement that we even went to the bariatric center to begin the Optifast program. Who does their first 5K at 67? My mom; My hero; That's who! I knew that this would change my race, as I usually run/ walk, and mom would only be walking, but that is OK – this is about finishing together. This time it was not just the two of us! My niece was running the race too. How cool was this? My 11-year-old niece, Alex, who was on the cross-country team, was doing her first Disney race! Three generations completing a race together. We may not have been in the first corral, we may not have crossed the finish line first, but it did not matter. We crossed and I cried tears of joy for my mom that day. SO DAMN PROUD OF HER! If you ever think you are too old to ever try something new, look to my mom…look to her for courage. I think she may have been bit by the race bug, as she has completed multiple races now. We may officially be considered back of the pack, but who cares? We are in the pack!

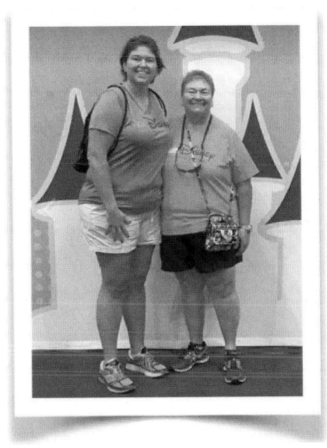

At the end of the race, my dad was there to greet us. Once again, Bobby-T, as I lovingly call him, caught a candid shot of me. When I finally made it back to the room, I started going through pictures and came across my picture in the same race, the year prior. I placed the pictures side-by-side of me completing the race in 2017 (left) and 2016 (right) There was an 80 pounds difference, but there was a much bigger difference. While I may look happy in both pictures, I was truly happy on the inside in 2017.

Clara Boyd

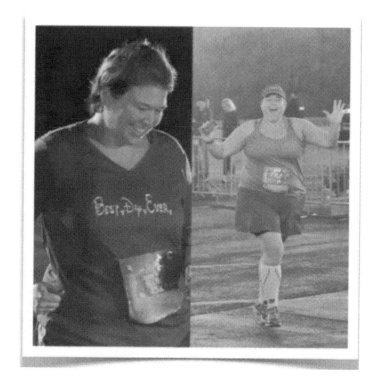

The next morning, I woke up at 3:30, but this time, it wasn't me that was racing. It was my sister's turn for her Disney race debut, a 10K to start. The running community is very supportive of each other, and we are very supportive of each other as a family, so even at 3:30 a.m., I will be her biggest fan. I knew getting up this early I would tired later on, but we planned to enjoy a few drinks at EPCOT. Being that tired I knew I would only be able to drink one maybe two before being done drinking, thus I would save money – winning all around! :) As we were on the bus to the start line, Kim confided in me that morning how proud of me she was that I had been running, and that I had inspired her to run. Are you kidding me? Here is my older sister that I have always looked up to, and she is telling me that I have inspired her? (yes Kim – I had to mention that you are older – love you!). I was speechless. I was so proud of her, and knew she was going to do great. Of course, she did. She finished strong! We were all there, the whole family, cheering her on at the finish line, ready to celebrate.

LETTING GO THROUGH MUSIC

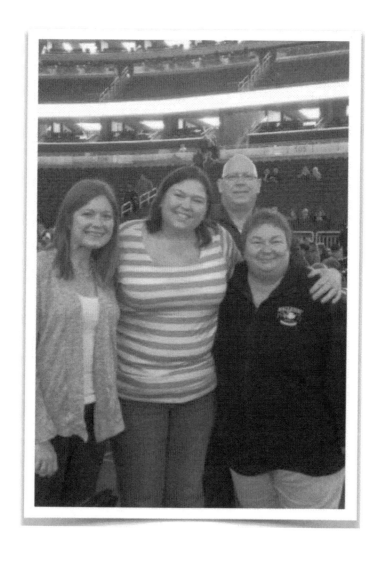

<u>The family at the Barry Manilow concert, 2014 - I loved that concert "Oh Mandy...."</u>

When you plan on running out your frustrations on the treadmill and you forget your ear buds. UGH! This is a great time to talk about technology. What did we do before technology? There are so many memes about people posting their exercise on social media. When I exercise, I have my Apple Watch with my Nike Run Club app on, with my wireless earbuds in my ears playing my play-set on my iPhone. I have self-diagnosed OCD. I need to my know my pace, my splits. Are they negative splits? If I am running in the morning before work, how many miles can I get in before I have to leave the gym? Don't forget the fact that my phone has an app for the treadmill that I am running on so it is tracking the calories I am burning, and another one that is paying me coins for every step I am taking. Did people really just get out there to run and be one with nature? I need to breathe… I need a little more namaste. Where is that hot yoga class when I need it? That ziplining??? I need to LET GO!

Music has always been an important part of my life. I was in multiple choirs as a child, and I twirled in the band. I even played piano for 6 years, although please do not even ask me to play chopsticks now (Sorry mom and dad for all of those lessons you paid for!). I associate music with memories, as I am sure many of us do. Growing up, my parents were good about introducing my sister and I to all different genres of music. If you play Barbara Streisand, Kenny Rogers, or Anne Murray, you might as well hand me a dust rag as this was the music we danced to as we cleaned the house. To this day, I get my best spring cleaning done to their music! I owe my love of musicals to my mom who would dance with Kim and me to Barbara Streisand's Broadway Album while we cleaned. My dad, was much more into Fleetwood Mac, Doobie Brothers, and Frankie Valli and the Four Seasons. Windows down singing at the top of our lungs to Doobie Brothers "Black Water" while driving with my dad, is one of my favorite memories growing up. It wasn't until I was in college that I said to my dad – I realize now why they are called the DOOBIE Brothers. I think on many levels he was happy it took until I was in college for me to understand the meaning of the band's name.

It is probably no surprise then that the music I listen to can directly affect my workout and the workout can affect the music I want to choose. I am an equal opportunity music lover – pop, top 40, country, everything other than techno. When it comes to running, I find Dave Matthews Band is what I love to run to, especially when I need my 30 minutes run in the mornings. Specifically, the *Crash* album. I know that there are DMB's meanings to the songs, and then there are my interpretations. But sometimes isn't music about what YOU get out of it? Let me take you through what I get out of this album.

"So Much to Say" – my warm up; get the kinks out.

"Two Step" – time to start running; alright Boyd pick up your pace.

"Crash Into Me" – 10 + minutes into the workout at this point. 6 + minutes into running. Don't crash. I know this song is about a peeping Tom, but I do like the vibe of it, especially at this point in the run. I am in a good flow, keep going Boyd, keep going.

"Too Much" – gluttonous attitude. Push it, Boyd. What have you been gluttonous about lately? Push it harder. DO NOT STOP NOW!

"41" – sing out loud – don't care at this point if anyone hears me. Hands are raised while singing. There have been so many interpretations of this song but one of them is about Dave Matthews being taken advantage of - an emotional split, if you will. Almost like the emotional split I am having with my weight that has controlled me my entire life. That is why I don't care who hears me sing this EVERY MORNING. ALMOST DONE RUNNING. FINISH STRONG BOYD!

"Say Goodbye" – during this song starts my cool down. It is slow enough to get your heart rate back down. 30 minutes done. Check the box and keep moving.

If I am not running, but working on hills, I listen to 90s R&B. Nothing like a little LL Cool J *Mr. Smith* to get you up that hill. It takes my mind off the fact that I am climbing, and it takes me back to Clemson, and my friends. We would drive around, listening to that CD for hours on a Friday night back in 1995/1996 before going out. While I was training for the 30-mile race, I listened to a lot of Olivia Newton-John and Billy Joel. Singing 1980s pop music will make training for a race go by quicker than you think!

Speaking of Billy Joel, two of his songs really helped me through the weight loss program - *Scenes from an Italian Restaurant*, and *Just the Way You Are*. They are still on my phone today. In my opinion, Billy Joel is one of the greatest American musicians ever. You may be scratching your head at this point, so let me explain. During the first part of Optifast, I had to drink shakes every 3 hours, and drink a certain amount of water daily. To help remind myself, I decided to set alarms on my phone. I got this idea from my mom. Of course, I did as she is a genius. *Just the Way You Are* was the alarm set for the shakes – I cannot think of a better song to hear as a confidence booster.

This was so powerful to me. I needed to be reminded multiple times daily I was loved JUST THE WAY I WAS. I have an amazing family and friends that love me no matter my size and I still needed that daily affirmation through this journey. I heard it from Billy Joel, well at least through my alarm. Every three hours, I got up, walked away from work or whatever I was doing and drank my shake; because I knew that was that was what was going to get me through the process. I decided to use the song *Just the Way You Are* as my morning alarm to make sure I started off my day the right way, and I still do to this day! It is a daily reminder that no matter what – I am loved just the way I am.

102

Clara Boyd

Scenes from an Italian Restaurant was set for the water. Well, if I could not drink a bottle of wine anymore, at least I could pretend all the water I was drinking was a bottle of wine. That alarm went off so much during the day, I was constantly drinking water. It is a habit I still continue to keep and it is rare that I drink anything other than water now.

It is amazing how music can influence so many aspects of your life, trigger memories, and provide inspiration on a daily basis. I still drive as often as I can with my windows down on the way home. The breeze in my face, blowing my troubles right out the window as I sing. Whether I sing along with Dave Matthews or the Doobie Brothers, the memories and great times come rushing back.

LETTING GO THROUGH PHYSICAL STRENGTH

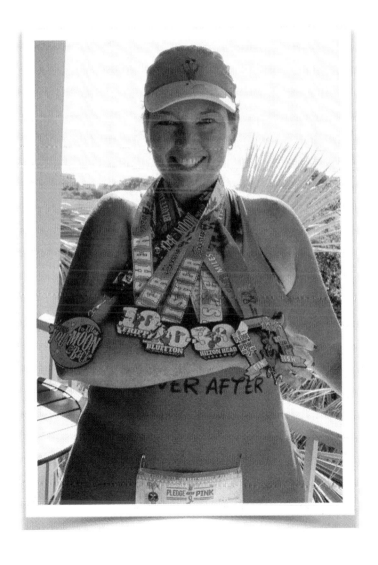

Clara Boyd

Two resolutions I am going to try to keep! I am writing 2 resolutions for 2018 - run 2018 miles (OK run/walk 2018 miles) and only drink good wine (OK - boxed wine counts.... ANY wine counts...hell - I'm in New Orleans - bring me a Hurricane)- HAPPY NEW YEAR to you and yours!!!! GO TIGERS. BEAT BAMA.

Two resolutions I am going to try to keep! I am writing this book in 2018, so we will see if this comes to fruition! If you follow football, you know my Clemson Tigers did not fare well in that game, but being a Clemson fan, I am loyal. Go Tigers! I am still on target for both of these resolutions. Both in moderation. 2018 miles in one year is equivalent to 5.55 miles per day, or 38.8 miles per week. Thank goodness I received the Apple watch for Christmas. It tracks my mileage so I do not need to.

Since the weight loss, alcohol consumption has been quite limited. I am allowed to drink; however, I look at it a lot differently now. In fact, I look at all food in a completely different way. Are those calories really worth it? How many miles will that rum runner equate to? How will I feel in the morning? Is it really worth it? My mindset used to be - I am indulging today, let me see if I can workout tomorrow. Then it went to – I am working out in the morning, I cannot indulge tonight.

Now it is, I am working out tomorrow, and I do not want to indulge tonight... I want to eat healthy to prepare for that workout. Do I still indulge? Yes, every so often. Do I still drink alcohol? Yes, in moderation. Am I a much cheaper date now? For sure.

January 7, 2018 – Facebook

Three notable/random thoughts about this week. #1 Found fifteen dollars in the laundry. Apparently, I am laundering money now. #2 I did not buy my Powerball tickets in New Hampshire. #3 Plugged in the computer - that must mean I get back to work officially again tomorrow. ***Bonus thought - I am on track with my 2018 miles in 2018!!!! 38 down many more to go!

January 27, 2018 – Facebook

Felt really good to get back to the gym after a 3-week hiatus because of sickness. Be healthy, but don't spread germs!!! Now to get in shape for Disney Princess!

Starting the year off with bronchitis really sucks, especially when you have a running goal. This is why I am all about getting ahead of pace. Now I am behind pace. But have no fear – I know I will make it up!

February 23, 2018 – Facebook

From the fairy Godmother, to Miles 1, 2, & 3, to beautiful sunrises, to Bob waking up early to cheer us on (BobbyT is the best!!!) Today is truly magical!

#rundisney — attending Disney Princess Half Marathon Weekend with Nancy and Laura at Walt Disney World.

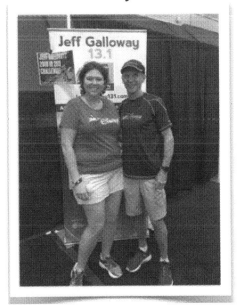

Clara Boyd

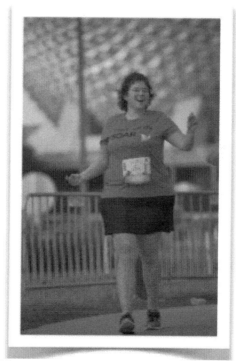

I told you I would become an expert at expo picture as well as race pictures!

I love these two pictures of me. If you remember, I spoke about Jeff Galloway earlier in the book. I could barely speak to him the first time I met him. Now I proudly speak to him as a fellow runner. I still respect him and his accomplishments, but I am so proud of my journey and each time we chat I update him. The second picture is me of course bopping to music. Who even knows what song was being played. I have no fear of singing in public. There is joy and celebration in this picture. The finish line was near, another race almost done, and celebrations were to be had!

March 3, 2018 – Facebook

Saturday. A day to sleep in. Somebody please tell my running addiction that.

Something happens physically when you change your lifestyle. Your body stops sleeping in. Sometimes this is a bad thing, but to me, this is good. When you sleep in, you are wasting the day away. You cannot get that time back! There is a gentleman at the gym that jokes with me in the morning. Mack always has three claps of encouragement and a smile on his face as we are the early birds on the treadmill. Whoever is the first one there, they will say to the other one, "The early bird gets the worm!" and this is so true - Go seize the morning…Go seize the day! You can always take a nap later. Naps are great! I love naps – and you can appreciate them so much more when everything you need to get done is already done.

March 15, 2018 – Facebook

Put the cognac in your coffee and lace up your shoes. No excuses. Let's get going.

I read the coolest story that day. It was about a woman named Ida Keeling. God bless this woman. Ida was 102 years old at the time of publication, drinks cognac in her coffee daily, and runs. Apparently, she had some stressors in her life and has found running to be her medicine. Ida broke many world records and is an inspiration to many. Many have called me an inspiration on my journey. Read Ida's story as she is a true inspiration – not me.

Everyone has stress but it is all about how you choose to handle it.

March 24, 2018 – Facebook

Distance: 3.11 miles

Time: 38:54

Pace: 12:30 min/mile

Thank you #Nike+ for reminding me. First sub 40 min 5K ever. Now to go conquer the day!

Clara Boyd

First sub 40 min 5K ever. It was 38 minutes and 54 seconds. For some people that is nothing. For me, that was everything! This is a great reminder that you are competing against yourself, and yourself only. My inspirational quote from Nike Run that day said – "Sometimes you run best on days when you did feel like running". I swear it was reading my mind – I did not want to get up that day. I must admit, I had not only plateaued my weight; I was climbing a little bit. The weekend prior was a college friend's wedding, and we celebrated hard. I indulged, and the scaled showed it. It was time to get serious again. So, for this to happen the first weekend of running, this was inspirational. Let's get after it.

This is a great time to talk about your support group. Who are your greatest supporters? Your cheerleaders? The people you can lean on when times are the toughest. When you cannot even believe in yourself, and you need someone else to believe in you. I have been lucky enough to have friends and family near and far that have always supported me in this journey. My dear friend Leigh, we talk multiple times per week and inevitably the conversation would lead to my weight loss journey. My girl, Robyn. While she may have been steps ahead of me during my races, literally and figuratively, she could physically push me like no one else. This princess taught me a lot about running and believing in yourself. About the time in the half marathon when I was feeling my lowest, I received that important text from Robyn. *"When your legs get tired…Run with you HEART!!"* I take this advice and use it in many aspects of my life. In my opinion, your heart is the strongest muscle in your body, and can be the most powerful. Run with your heart, and you will be running in the right direction!

It is great to go on a journey with others. Remember on the very first page of the book I spoke of how no two people will ever be on the same journey – no matter how similar the itinerary may look. Perhaps they are in the same car, listening to the same song, looking at the same foliage on the side of the road. However, their experiences will be different. This doesn't mean that you have to go at it alone. Having someone there with you makes the journey exciting, or maybe just endurable. Sometimes their journey is not as long as yours, or maybe their journey will parallel yours, but you still can be each other's support systems. From a coworker, to friends that live near and far, to family members, there are people in my life that have been with me every step of the way on this journey. Sometimes it included sharing the same meal plan, workout clothes, or even conversation. There have been people that have been on this journey with me who live in the same city and speak daily, while others were states away, and we communicated solely online or on the phone.

Nowadays with technology, there are so many opportunities to hold your friends accountable and challenge each other. When you have someone with common goals, it makes it eas- ier to stay accountable. I have enjoyed watching friends and family members start their weight loss journeys and achieve their goals! Their support for my journey means everything to me, and I hope they know, I am always there to support them…ALWAYS!

April 12, 2018 – Facebook

Oh Bon Jovi - Late for my workout this morning. But I was able to hear my Jersey boys serenade me on the way. Not a shabby way to start my day!!!!

Hello Bon Jovi!!! Being a Jersey Girl, the songs of Bon Jovi or Springsteen just does it for me. While I grew up in Florida, I was born in Jersey, remember. You can take the girl out of Jersey, but you can NEVER take the Jersey out of the girl! It is interesting how my music on the way to the gym will set my mood at the gym. Listening to *Bed of Roses*, I ended up walking hills very calmly. The next day, I heard LL Cool J *Mama Said Knock You Out* on the way to the gym and had one of the best intervals run with weight lifting sessions following.

May 3, 2018 – Facebook

Clara Boyd

As I am exhausted this morning dragging myself out of bed to start my first of two workouts this morning I have hit the 90-pound weight loss mark. I am so close to 100 pounds lost, that goal is in sight. If you think that I'm stopping now, get the heck out of my way! Here's to soon hitting 100 pounds lost, and soon being into ONE-derland again :) Happy Thursday to you, make it a great day!

Some days even after losing 90 pounds, it is hard to find an intrinsic reward to get out of bed. And then you get on the scale and you see that number 236. Can I really be only 10 pounds away from hitting 100 pounds lost? What does that even look like? I cannot even fathom that! That to me is motivation.

<u>July 8, 2018 – Facebook</u>

How Clara Got Her Groove Back. Kind of sounds like the title to a movie. I will admit it. While texting a friend this week while gossiping after having a glass of wine, I said - I am getting my groove back. And for those of you that know a certain movie, **wink wink***...*

As I look back on the last 600 days (yes - it has been exactly 600 days since this journey started) I realize that this has not just been a physical journey but an emotional journey as well. 100 pounds lost. ONE HUNDRED POUNDS LOST!!! What a great week to officially hit this goal, as this Friday, I turn 42. I do not say this for the accolades of my birthday, but the celebration of this journey. So, while we may not be in Jamaica to celebrate this week, Cape Cod will suit just fine!

There are milestones and memories in there that were public and private. Some that made me laugh and made me cry. There are physical things that are embarrassing that come with 100 pounds weight loss like sagging skin - I am all about getting skin removal surgery now! But there are greater physical benefits including my blood work- it has never looked better in my adult life! Please know from the start... Every pound has meaning to me. Everyone was just as important before the 100-pound mark. 11-pound mark - first week at the Bariatric Center.

Losing One Hundred Pounds

27 pounds - I weighed 299 - never to see 300s ever again. 67 pounds - brain surgery. 85 pounds – officially declared free from sleep apnea - things you don't forget, and major milestones.

Many of you know my story so I will not regurgitate it. But what you may not know... There are days that I still feel like the girl that weighed 326 pounds and do not feel that I have lost a pound; and then there are days I see pictures of myself at that weight and get physically sick looking at the pictures.

At the 40-pound mark, I could not see a difference. I was in different clothes, and my blood work was amazing, but I could not see anything yet. A friend's husband, who I see once every few years, took forty pounds of frozen ground beef out of the freezer and placed it on the kitchen counter and said - "That is what you have lost - right there". Talk about eye opening. That is what I needed to see. I think of that day often. When I walk through the grocery store, I keep wanting to ask the butcher what 100 pounds of meat looks like. The butcher would probably think I was crazy!

I skipped my 20-year high school reunion. Paid for it. Never went. Too embarrassed to go. Thanks to social media, everyone knew what I looked like already, but I could not face any- one knowing that I weighed 326 pounds. I was actually interviewing for a position at work that week (that was the excuse I gave), but it was less than a two-hour drive back to my home town from the interview. I could have made it. Did not go. What sucks is a friend of mine from high school died this past year. Hadn't seen him in years, and because of my embarrassment, I did not see him when I had the chance. I will be there for my 25th.

When I went on my first cruise, I was too heavy to even go down the slide (before I started losing weight). There was a weight limit. I lied to my nieces saying my foot really hurt me something awful, and so I did not want to climb the stairs. In reality, I was scared being 26 pounds over the weight limit - would I get stuck in the tube or would the slide hold me as it went out over the water??? My second cruise was to Alaska, I weighed 250 pounds when we boarded. I was able to zip line and participate in all activities. I could comfortably sit in the seats on the plane. I was starting to feel like a human being again and not someone that was having to sit on the sidelines and watch everyone else enjoy life.

With this weight loss comes an interesting emotional concern that I did not see coming. In my mind, I am no longer a wallflower. When I was 326 pounds, I could be as loud and outspoken as I wanted to be. Because people were not going to notice me for any reason other than being loud. There was a wall up, and I was guarded. Quite comfortable with it. The wall is coming down now, and that scares me. I am vulnerable now. Quiet and reserved at times. I receive compliments and I honestly do not know how to accept them. I usually make excuses, or brush them off, hoping to be in the background. I have received compliments my whole life. I have been surrounded by people that love me - truly love me my whole life, and for that I am grateful. But I have never heard the compliments and taken them to heart - until this journey. A quote I read tonight went something like this - "You've always been beautiful. But now you are just choosing to be healthy, fit, powerful, and strong." I like that attitude towards compliments and beauty. Unfortunately, on this journey I have met some roadblocks, be it people in my life or other obstacles. There are people with their own agendas who did not want me to succeed. That is OK...my goal was bigger than their agenda. Their agenda really had nothing to do with me, and I know that. I choose not to focus on them. I have chosen to focus on the people that have been my greatest supporters. There are people that are in my life daily that keep me focused. Plan out my meals with me, down to the times and portions. Make sure I have done my two workouts in the morning. Making sure every decision I make is a positive one towards my goals. You know who you are. You know I would not hit this goal without you. YOU keep me accountable. You know I love you. Thank You. (And yes - I have stayed accountable on vacation - Val made sure of it!)

There are friends and family that check in with me, be it daily, weekly, or whenever they can. Each one of these people are the reason I hit this goal. I did not do this on my own.

Then there are the friends that reach out to say I inspire them. (Please note - I am literally crying as I write this) I am humbled every time I hear this. I took this journey out of necessity. I was scared I was going to have a heart attack in my early 40s. My life was spinning out of control. And now I am being called an inspiration? I am speechless. So, when someone calls me inspiring, all I can truly and humbly say is, Thank You. So many that have admitted to me that I am their inspiration - I have yet to tell them that THEY were the inspiration for me to run, to workout, to keep going. This journey is hard and in no way could be done alone. There were many days that I did not want to work out or to continue on this journey, and then would see a post from someone, and that was all I needed to lace up my shoes and go for a run.

The Bariatric doctor who works closely with me believes that my goal weight is 208 pounds. So, this journey is not over. I would like to see 198, just to see "one-derland" again. This journey will never be over. The latest research in peer-reviewed medical journals show that obesity really is a disease. It is more than just "putting down the sandwich"; I say that because there is a chemical change within your brain when you become obese that wants your body to go back to your highest weight. That is why many people gain the weight back. People go back to their old habits and their body holds onto those calories very quickly. I am on two medicines currently to help trick my brain to stop want- ing to revert back to the high weight. Please do not think that I am on "diet pills" and that is how I am losing weight. I work out for 1.5-2 hours daily including running and weight training and eat quite healthy. Once I am at my goal weight, it will take approximately two years for my brain to realize that I should not weigh 326 pounds. This will be a lifestyle change for the rest of my life.

Two years ago, I could barely fit through a doorway; and today when I am running, or looking in the mirror while lifting weights, I envision that 326-pound girl, and know I will never be her again. Yesterday morning while working out I could see the curves in my collarbone and the muscles in my neck every time I came up on a crunch. Lord knows the last time I could see my collarbones. My physical fitness challenge

Clara Boyd

this year for myself is the barre classes - so you better be ready!

I am focusing on the positives in life now - I may not be Stella (or have Angela Bassett's killer shoulders!) ... but I am sure as hell getting my groove back!

LETTING GO IS A CONSCIOUS EFFORT

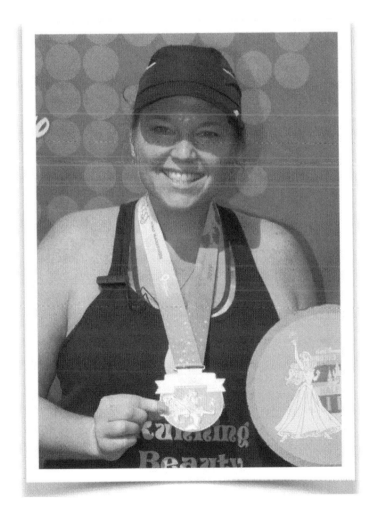

When I wrote the post on July 8th I had so many people reach out to me publicly, but even more privately. They spoke about how much they could relate and the emotional struggle that weight gain could bring. Many were going through the same journey themselves, others were hoping to one day join me on this journey. Some were saying I was an inspiration. Once again – I am humbled. If nothing else, this journey has left me a very humbled person.

When you lose weight, there are some things they don't tell you. The physical one is that this is the only addiction in the world that people actually have to live with. This is something I will face the rest of my life.

Eating out can be challenging if you do not prepare, but if you do, it can be kind of fun – you just have to be adventurous. Look at the menu online before going to the restaurant will help make sure you can find something suitable. Waiters and waitresses really don't care as long as you tip them. I have yet to order directly off a menu since I have lost weight as there is some sort of change to my order. Double veggies; steamed, not fried – some healthy change to the menu item. Remember, it is okay to change your order and don't feel guilty or embarrassed, feel empowered! You are making better choices for yourself. If the staff informs you it is not possible, inform them that you are not interested in eating there. Find power in yourself. I have walked out of a restaurant before, it is okay.

Being single, of course, has its benefits when eating at home. I don't keep a lot of food in my house. If it is not in my house, I do not have the temptation to eat it. My niece and I ran errands the other day including going to the grocery store to pick up a few items. As we walked up and down each aisle talking about her day at school, catching up on all the 7th grade gossip, she pushed the cart. She was loading the grocery cart with what I was asking her to put in there. By the end of the store there were 3 cases of water and 4 pints of Halo ice cream. (They were BOGO, and will last me about a month.) She looked at me and said – "No wonder you are single. There is nothing in your refrigerator." Sigh – out of the mouths of babes.

Another thing I was not prepared for - you are going to lose your identity. I always identified as the fat sidekick friend, and so that was the role I have always played. Now, I don't know who I am; I don't know how to act, how to take a compliment. It sounds silly but I am 42 years old and get embarrassed when someone compliments me. I talked about it in the prior Facebook post, and it still rings true today. It is something I work on daily – an insecurity that has surfaced with losing weight. Others have confided to me the same about themselves, which got me thinking – how many people have such insecurities and hide it so well? Here I am, writing a book about the fact I have lost 100+ pounds, screaming it on social media, and I am insecure? Yes, I am. Where do I go from here? Who do I identify as now?

Who do I identify as after I finish losing the weight? I will have a whole new journey – how exciting!

Speaking of identities, can we talk about social media identities and real life? How many people have their social life identity and then their real-life identity? You know those peo- ple – where everything is rainbows and sunshine on social media – they just went and ran a marathon, and did not even break a sweat, baked the perfect batch of cookies for their per- fect children who have the perfect grades, have the perfect husband, and the perfect house? Then in reality – their entire life is falling apart. Sometimes social media is not the place to make yourself feel better. You scroll through these posts and you think what are they doing so right and here I sit with the dishes in the sink, the laundry on the second cycle through the dryer because it is easier than ironing out the wrinkles. My kid was in detention at school, and my husband is not the top salesman of the month. Guess what? THAT is real life! And that is a-OK! Because that is reality. One of my favorite clichés is that is the grass is greener in the other side. I like to add my additional thought to it... The other side is fertilized with bull. Remember that many social media posts are just that. You are on your own journey, and never need to compare yourself to anyone else, especially on social media. The posts throughout this journey have been unfiltered, unlike pictures on social media. Remember my friends, you are beautiful – just the way you are!

Reality is also that there are going to be setbacks. I have had setbacks on this journey; with my weight and with my physical and emotional gains. January 1st is not the only day to re-start your journey. Every day is a new chance to hit reset. Journaling was the perfect way to let go of emotional anxieties. Once I could see past the anxiety of the weight loss and the accompanying benefits, there was a sense of self-esteem and assurance that I could continue – even through the plateaus, setbacks, and struggles. When those setbacks happen, reading the journal entries, reaching out to friends, or looking at old pictures of where I started was would get me started right back on the journey.

LETTING GO OF EVERYTHING

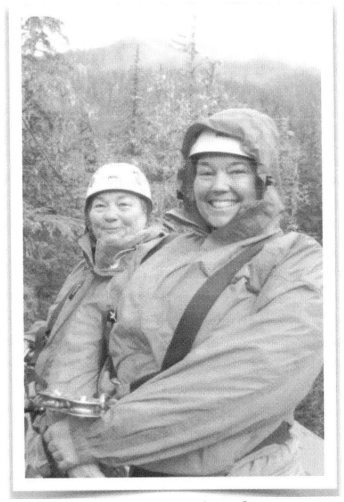

There are so many quotes out there about fear, none more famous in my opinion than FDR's "The only thing we have to fear, is fear itself." I think back to Alaska, when I was so fearful to let go of that first zip-line platform. What was I so fearful of that day? Why could I not let go of my fears? What were my fears with losing weight? Was I waiting until something went wrong? Why was I always putting others before myself? I did fear the changes that would come with losing weight, but I am courageous enough to admit it. There are aspects of my life that I have held onto for too long, fearing change. During my annual trip this past summer up to Cape Cod, Val had a heart-to-heart with me on my birthday. What did I want to change about my life? Was I okay with how things were going? Did I want things to change? I was feeling complacent with some things in my life, and I knew I was forgetting about someone again. ME. Why do the best conversations always involve Dunkin Donuts coffee? As I sat there that morning, tears dripping into my coffee, knowing it was time to let go of fear, and time for change. Time to put ME first again. I lost sight of ME. 42 was MY year.

Upon my return home, my first weigh in at the bariatric center, the therapist called me back from the waiting room to weigh me. Talk about divine intervention. Typically, it is a nurse or the nutritionist – rarely do I get the therapist who calls me back for weigh me. She asked about my trip, excited to hear all about it, and I told her about my conversation with Val. She listened, and then gently reminded me that relationships will change after transformation. People that you need in your life, before and during the transformation, to be your rock, may not be the same after the transformation - and that it is okay. They may need to take a different role in your life after the transformation; do not feel guilty about it. Let them go. I needed to hear that. There are so many people that have helped me through this journey that I could never repay for their support emotionally and physically. I also need to live for me. That includes finding me.

After reading the January 30, 2017 Facebook entry, a dear friend of mine, yet again – another sister from another mister, Vivian encouraged me to take all of these journals entries and write a book. I knew many people had watched my transformation both in person and online. I recognized that I was inspiring people, but I did not know the extent. I knew after the conversation with Val that this was how I was going to live for myself again, how I would put myself first. Writing this book is letting go of fear, letting go of guilt of being overweight. I would have never had the courage to do this at 326 pounds. The 326-pound wallflower, who thought no one noticed her unless she was loud and obnoxious, who was the life of the party, would not have let people into the inner circle of her life like this. I know now I needed let go of the anger I had of people telling me how to live my life. I NEEDED to let go the guilt I felt about putting myself first.

At the beginning of my writing, my intention was to specifically write about the weight loss. By the second day of outlining the book, I recognized quickly that this journey encompasses more than just the numbers on the scale. This journey is not only physical, but mental, spiritual and emotional as well. It is about living life, overcoming fears, and challenging myself. During one of the final days of the writing process, I found myself a little stressed, and decided to take a break to do yoga. During the final phase called shavasana, meaning corpse pose, is a deep relaxation time. The instructor talked about surrendering and letting go. For most, this would allow them to relax, for me – it was a sign to finish strong! I needed to get back to work to finish LETTING GO!

Challenge yourself. Run YOUR race. Take on that hot yoga class. Get on the plane. Go on vacation. Live outside of your comfort zone.

This is ME jumping off the zipline platform of life - eyes wide open, arms and legs extended, letting go of my inhibitions, my fears, my insecurities. This me exhaling. This is me, living life. Out loud, finding peace in LETTING GO ~ Clara

Clara Boyd

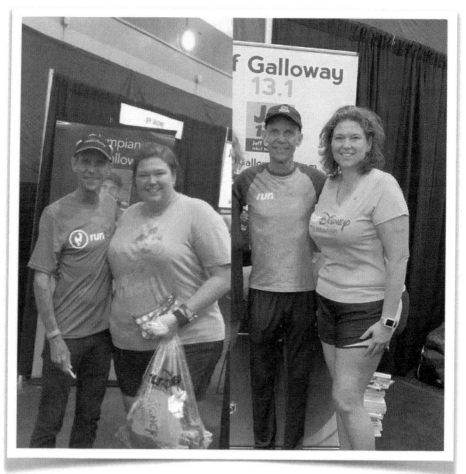

Jeff Galloway and me in Fall of 2015 and again in Spring of 2019

REFERENCES & PHOTOGRAPGY ACKNOWLEDGEMENTS

Perry, Susan. "Obese Women Experience Much More Negative Social Stigma than Previously Thought, Study Finds." MinnPost, 15 Mar. 2016, www.minnpost.com/second-opinion/2016/01/obese-women-experience-much-more-negative-social-stigma-previously-thought-st/.

Photo of me - Sarasota High School. The Sailors Log, 1992. Print.

Photo of Ann Scott, Photo courtesy of Barbara Clark. https://flgov.smugmug.com/FirstLadyAnnScott/August-2018/8-7-2018-FLVS/

Once again, as mentioned in the "My Thoughts" portion of this book, at the time of press, I am not a spokesman for any of the products mentioned in this book. This includes, but is not limited to the following: OPTIFAST which is registered trademark of Société des Produits Nestlé S.A., Vevey, Switzerland., Sparkle Skirts, Jeff Galloway.com, Dave Matthews Band, Barry Manilow, LL Cool J, Billy Joel, Barbara Streisand, Doobie Brothers, Frankie Valli and the Four Seasons, Kenny Rogers, Anne Murray, Fleetwood Mac, Nike, Apple, Pledge the Pink, Dunkin Donuts, runDisney & Walt Disney World which are affiliated with the Walt Disney Company. I personally think that these are all great products and performers for my personal needs, but please make choices that are right for you and your personal health needs. Please seek advice from your medical professionals.

Made in the
USA
Columbia, SC